W9-CDM-791

DISCARD

ENCYCLOPEDIA OF
FAMILY HEALTH

THIRD EDITION

ENCYCLOPEDIA OF
FAMILY HEALTH

——THIRD EDITION——

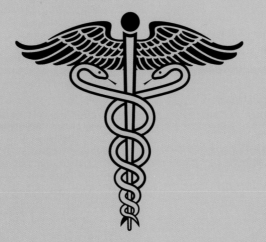

CONSULTANTS

David B. Jacoby, M.D.
Johns Hopkins School of Medicine

Robert M. Youngson, M.D.
Royal Society of Medicine

VOLUME 17

ULCERS — ZEST

MARSHALL CAVENDISH
New York · London · Singapore

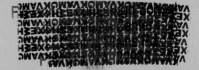

MEDICAL CONSULTANTS

Second Edition
David B. Jacoby, M.D.
Johns Hopkins School of Medicine
Associate Professor of Pulmonary and Critical
    Care Medicine

Third Edition
Robert M. Youngson, M.D.
Fellow of the Royal Society of Medicine
Officer of the Order of St John of Jerusalem
Diploma in Tropical Medicine and Hygiene
Fellow of the Royal College of Ophthalmologists

CONTRIBUTORS TO THIRD EDITION

David Arnot   Tom Jackson
Deborah Evans   Nathan Lepora
Leon Gray   Fiona Plowman
Joanna Griffin   Alison Tarrant
Tim Harris   Aruna Vasudevan
John Jackson

Picture Credits
(b – bottom; t – top; r – right; l – left; c – center)

Cover: Digital Vision: c; Dynamic Graphics: John Foxx & Images 4
Communication b/l, b/r; PhotoDisc: Don Farrall b/c, Keith Brofsky t/r.

Alan Hutchinson Library: 2351, 2358, 2371l, 2424b/l; Argentum: 2130; ARS:
Keith Weller 2356t/r, Peggy Greb 2356b, 2379, Scott Bauer 2352, 2353,
2354b/r; Biophoto Associates: 2329b, 2334, 2350all, 2369t, 2424b/r, 2428r,
2433r, 2438; Bridgeman Art Library: 2397; Brown Reference Group: 2445r; C
James Webb: 2311t, 2311b, 2420c/r, 2421c/r, 2434b; Charles Day: 2312r,
2435; Colorific: 2349l, Neil Leifer/Sports Illustrated 2318; Corbis: Cat Gwynn
2401, David Turnley 2425l, Duomo 2422, George Disario 2419, Georgina
Bowater 2436, James Marshall 2416, Karl Weatherly 2403, Kevin Fleming 2339,
Lawrence Manning 2398, Lester V Bergman 2313, 2437b/r, Patrick Bennett
2337, Richard T Nowitz 2400, Ricki Rosen 2346t, Roy Morsch 2364, Shepard
Sherbell 2349, Steve Prezant 2394, Terry Whittaker/FLPA 2402; Corbis Sygma:
Aim Patrice 2406; Daimler Chrysler: 2410; Di Lewis: 2373, 2375, 2383;
Dynamic Graphics: John Foxx & Images 4 Communication 2367, 2409; Empics:
SportsChrome 2424t; Fotomax Index: 2358; Getty Images: 2331b, 2347,
2365t, 2382, 2387, 2446, Petrified Collection 2411; Graham Strong: 2354t,
2354b/l; Health Education Council: 2331t; Heather Angel: 2421t/c;
Imagingbody.com: 2324, 2357t, 2413, 2437b/l; Institute of Dermatology:
2312l, 2344, 2388, 2396b, 2437t/l; John Watney: 2328, 2362, 2396t/l; John
Wright: 2439; Kobal Collection: 2418; London Scientific Fotos: 2421c/l,
2421b/r; Mary Evans Picture Library: 2390; N Shah FRCS: 2389; PHIL: 2325b,
2372; PhotoDisc: Don Tremain 2385, Scott T Baxter 2361, 2430; Photos.com:
2332t/l, 2355t, 2355b, 2356t/l, 2395; Popperfoto: 2445l; Rex Features: 2326,
2427, Action Press 2423t, AGB Photo Library 2425r, Alix/Phanie 2332b, David
Buchan 2426, Eastlight 2330, Garo/Phanie 2315, Lehtikuva Oy/Airio 2414,
Neale Haynes 2429, Phanie Agency 2417, Richard Gardener 2332t/r, SAI
2317t/r, 2317c/r, Sipa Press 2408, 2428l, SXW 2440; Robert Harding: 2325t,
2359, 2392, 2412; Ron Sutherland: 2343, 2421b/l, 2442all, 2443all, 2444all;
Spectrum: 2380; Science Photo Library: 2336, 2346b, 2357b, 2370, 2371r,
Alexander Tsiaras 2319, David Gifford 2322, Geoff Tompkinson 2338, Hank
Morgan 2341t, John Greim 2320t, Lawrence Mulvehill 2316, 2317t/l, Professor
J James 2314, Richard T Nowitz 2320b, Sheila Terry 2405, Stevie Grand 2360;
Syndication International: 2433l, 2433c; Vision International: 2369b, CNRI
2431, 2434t/l, 2434t/r; Westminster Medical School: 2341b; Zefa: 2423b.

Marshall Cavendish
99 White Plains Road
Tarrytown, NY 10591-9001

www.marshallcavendish.com

Library of Congress Cataloging-in-Publication Data

Encyclopedia of family health / David B. Jacoby, Robert M. Youngson.--
3rd ed.
        p. cm.
Includes bibliographical references and index.
    ISBN 0-7614-7486-2 (set)
    ISBN 0-7614-7503-6 (vol 17)
1. Medicine, Popular--Encyclopedias. 2. Health--Encylopedias. 1. Jacoby, David
B. II. Youngson, R. M. III. Marshall Cavendish Corporation. IV. Title
RC81.A2E5 2004
610'.3--dc22   2003065554

Printed in China
08 07 06 05 04 5 4 3 2 1

Marshall Cavendish

Editor: Joyce Tavolacci
Editorial Director: Paul Bernabeo
Production Manager: Alan Tsai

The Brown Reference Group

Project Editor: Anne Hildyard
Editors: Jane Lanigan, Sally McFall
Designers: Jeni Child, Reg Cox, Karen Frazer
Picture Researcher: Clare Newman
Indexer: Kay Ollerenshaw
Illustrations: Samantha J. Elmhurst
Managing Editor: Tim Cooke
Art Director: Dave Goodman

This encyclopedia is not intended for use as a substitute for advice, consultation, or treatment by a licensed medical practitioner. The reader is
advised that no action of a medical nature should be taken without
consultation with a licensed medical practitioner, including action that
may seem to be indicated by the contents of this work, since individual
circumstances vary and medical standards, knowledge, and practices
change with time. The publishers, authors, and medical consultants
disclaim all liability and cannot be held responsible for any problems
that may arise from use of this encyclopedia.

CONTENTS

KEY TO COLOR CODING OF ARTICLES

HUMAN BODY

DISEASES AND OTHER DISORDERS

TREATMENTS AND CURES

PREVENTION AND DIAGNOSIS OF DISEASE

HUMAN BEHAVIOR

Ulcers

Although commonly affecting the stomach or duodenum, ulcers also occur elsewhere on the body. Caused by a variety of factors, from disease to injury, they can range from a mild irritation to a serious condition.

Questions and Answers

My teenage daughter keeps getting ulcers on her forearm, and our doctor says that he believes she is inflicting the injuries on herself. How can this be?

The doctor probably suspects that your daughter is suffering from a psychological condition, the symptom of which is self-mutilation. Self-inflicted injury may be performed to gain attention or avoid some anxiety-producing situation at home or school and she may be unaware that she is injuring herself. Ask your doctor about taking her to have psychiatric counseling.

I have an embarrassing ulcer in my groin region. What could this be due to?

There are a number of possible causes of an ulcer in the groin, ranging from mild irritation or injury to more serious sexually transmitted diseases. See your doctor as soon as possible to have the cause of the ulcer diagnosed.

My father is bedridden and suffers from bedsores. How can these be prevented?

A special air mattress, which has sections that can be alternately inflated and deflated to change the pressure-bearing areas, will help considerably. Also, always ensure that his position in bed is changed at frequent intervals.

Do ulcers in the mouth indicate that one is run-down or unhealthy?

Not necessarily. Mouth ulcers can be caused by a number of different factors. Recurrent ulcers caused by herpes are particularly common and often appear following any emotional stress or during illness. However, mouth ulcers may also be a symptom of anemia, and if this is the case, one would feel run-down.

An ulcer is a localized area of loss of tissue on the surface of the skin or on any other surface in the body, such as the wet lining of the digestive tract and other internal surfaces. The result of such loss is an open sore. An ulcer heals slowly because its edges are separated, and healing can occur only by growth of tissue in from the edges. Ulcers are usually associated with inflammation somewhere in the body (see Inflammation). Loss of surface tissue as a result of a wound from injury is not primarily an ulcer, but if infection occurs such a wound may become ulcerated (see Wounds).

Ulcers are often circular or oval in shape and sometimes irregular in outline. Ulcers on the surface of the body vary considerably in their depth, some involving skin loss only, but others extending deep into the muscle or bone beneath the skin. The causes of ulcers are numerous and range from a mild irritation or injury to a serious disease.

Mouth and lip ulcers

Mouth ulcers are a common problem, and occur either as a onetime condition or as a recurrent disease. Almost everyone has at some time or other suffered the discomfort of the nonrecurrent type of mouth ulcers. They are brought on by a variety of factors but are usually due to some identifiable physical, chemical, or biological cause or are a symptom of some underlying condition.

Physical causes of mouth ulceration include irritation from jagged teeth, compulsive cheek-chewing, too vigorous use of a toothbrush, and burning from hot foods or drinks (see Burns). Chemical causes include caustic drugs, tablets, and sweets that are allowed to dissolve in the

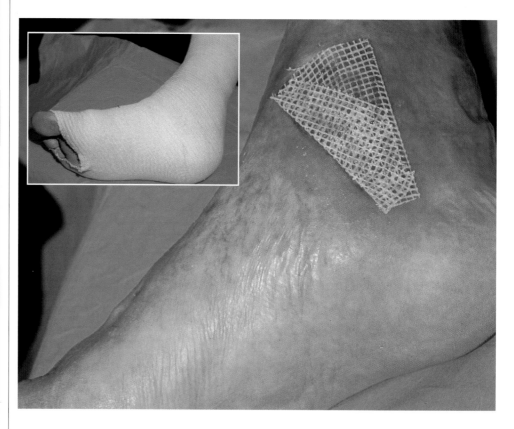

▲ *A leg ulcer is first cleaned, covered with a sterile gauze pad cut to fit, padded for protection, and then bandaged so that even pressure is applied to the wound.*

mouth; strong antiseptics; and mouthwashes and chemicals used in dental treatment.

Biological causes of ulcers include the syphilis bacterium, various fungi, and the herpes simplex virus. A syphilitic chancre in the mouth is rare but, like a chancre anywhere, is very serious. It is sexually acquired, consisting of a single round, button-sized, painless ulcer on the tongue or lip (see Tongue).

By contrast, an acute herpes infection in the mouth consists of numerous smaller, painful ulcers on the gums, tongue, and membranes that line the inside of the cheeks or the inside of the lips (see Cold Sores; Gums and Gum Diseases).

Nonrecurrent, but persistent, mouth ulcers may also be a symptom of diabetes, blood diseases, or tuberculosis (see Blood; Diabetes; Tuberculosis). Cancer of the lip, though uncommon, often makes its first appearance as an ulcer.

Aphthous ulcers

"Aphthous ulcer" is the medical term given to a condition of mouth inflammation characterized by intermittent episodes of painful mouth ulcers on the internal mucous

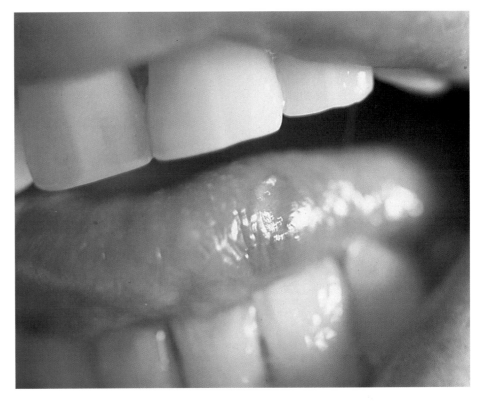

▲ *The aphthous ulcer, seen here on the tongue, is the most common of all single mouth ulcers and can be caused by broken teeth or spicy food.*

membrane. Aphthous ulcers are also known as canker sores, aphthous stomatitis, or ulcerative stomatitis. These ulcers are covered with a grayish discharge. They are surrounded by a red halo, and occur singly or in groups. Even without treatment aphthous ulcers will heal spontaneously in one to two weeks.

Recurrent mouth ulcers affect about one person in three. They usually consist of numerous small, painful ulcers on or inside the lips,

or on the tongue, throat, or roof of the mouth, and may persist for a week or two, disappear, and then appear again some weeks or months later. The causes of recurrent mouth ulcers are not so well understood, but it is known that those confined to the lips are nearly always due to the herpes simplex virus. Those inside the mouth may also be caused by herpes, but are more likely due to an allergy, a nutritional deficiency, anemia, or celiac disease (see Allergies; Anemia; Celiac Disease).

▼ *Habitual cheek-biting can become so self-destructive as to cause a line of tissue breakdown that soon leads to an ulcer.*

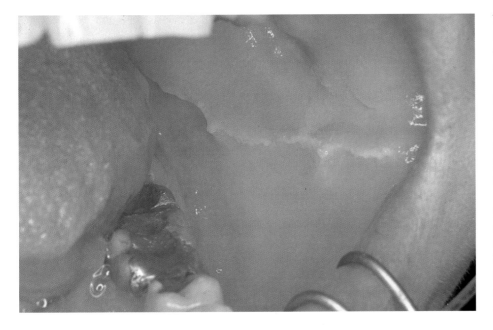

Mouth ulcers and general disease

Mouth ulcers may provide clues to the presence of many other general diseases. They are, for instance, regular features of several important and potentially dangerous disorders such as ulcerative colitis, Behçet's disease, and Reiter's syndrome.

Ulcerative colitis is an inflammatory disease of unknown cause affecting the lower part of the large intestine and the rectum. There is extensive ulceration of the inner lining of the intestine, leading to the passage of blood and mucus in the stools and episodes of constipation.

Behçet's disease is characterized by recurrent simultaneous or successive attacks of mouth and genital ulcers and an internal and inflammatory disorder of the eyes known as uveitis. The disease affects men more often than women, and occurs most often in adolescence. The uveitis is by far the more serious aspect of the disorder. This calls

Questions and Answers

My mother has a leg ulcer, and the doctor has told her that she should sleep with the foot of her bed raised up. Why is this necessary?

Your mother is almost certainly suffering from a type of leg ulcer that develops from varicose veins. In this condition, blood tends to pool in the lower legs. Fluid collects and eventually the skin in the area becomes thinned and breaks down to form an ulcer. During treatment it helps for the person to keep the leg raised above the body during sleep or rest, thereby encouraging normal blood circulation.

Is it possible to have a stomach ulcer without knowing it?

Certainly. Many people accept that a small amount of indigestion is normal. A fair proportion of these people would be found to have an active ulcer, or the signs of an old ulcer, if they had a gastroscopy. If the ulcer is asymptomatic (without any symptoms) and does not have any complications, then it is really not a great concern.

I've been told that I have to eat frequently because of a stomach ulcer. Now I'm putting on a lot of weight. What can I do about this?

The trick is to eat frequent small meals. The idea is that frequent small meals do not allow the level of acid to build up, since the acid is continually being neutralized by the food. Obviously, you do risk putting on weight, and you should aim to eat a normal amount of food, but split it into a greater number of smaller meals.

Does surgery for a stomach ulcer leave a huge, ugly scar?

No, because minimally invasive surgery is increasingly used. This type of surgery leaves four or five tiny scars which are barely visible after a few months. Other advantages are a shorter hospital stay, less postoperative pain, and reduced recovery time.

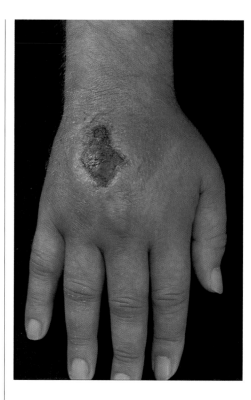

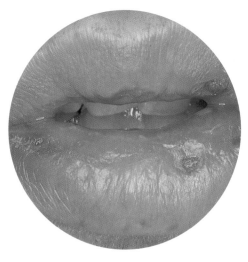

▲ *Herpes is often the cause of clusters of small ulcers on the lips, a condition that is also known as gingivostomatitis.*

◄ *This ulcer was caused by a faulty IV drip attached to the hand. An anticancer drug accidentally leaked out onto the skin.*

for skilled ophthalmic management if permanent impairment to the eyesight is to be avoided (see Eyes and Eyesight; Ophthalmology).

Reiter's syndrome is also associated with internal eye inflammation. The syndrome consists of mouth and genital ulcers, and inflammation of the urine outlet tube (see Urethra) with discharge, uveitis, and joint inflammation (see Arthritis). Many cases may also involve persistent diarrhea. These different elements may occur together or separately at intervals of months or years, but once the arthritis is established it is often continuously present.

The treatment of any mouth ulcer depends greatly on the cause; for example, dental therapy for jagged or decayed teeth, surgery for lip cancer, and a gluten-free diet for celiac disease. In many cases of recurrent ulceration, when the exact cause cannot be found, mouthwashes, tablets, and analgesic creams and jellies are often prescribed by the doctor to help soothe the pain. Herpetic ulcers are treated with the drug aciclovir (Zovirax) formulated as a cream, which should be applied at the earliest indication of symptoms and repeated about five times a day.

When an ulcer becomes persistent, or when there are repeated bouts of ulcers, it is extremely important for a person to visit his or her doctor to have the cause diagnosed. A strong mouthwash or gargle may seem the most likely method of treating a mouth ulcer, but the solution of the mouthwash may be strong enough to aggravate the condition. In addition, the underlying cause will remain untreated. So it is essential to seek medical advice immediately.

Leg ulcers

Like mouth ulcers, leg ulcers are quite common and have a number of different causes: injury, infection, blood disease (such as sickle-cell anemia), and cancer are frequent causes (see Cancer; Sickle-Cell Anemia). The most common cause, however, is disease of the blood vessels in the legs.

Blocked or narrow arteries (see Arteries and Artery Disease) diminish the blood supply to the tissues, causing the tissues to die and break down, thereby producing an ulcer. Ulcers of this type tend to occur on the lower leg or foot, and have a regular appearance. They may be several inches wide, may be quite deep, and are extremely painful.

Defective valves in the veins not only cause varicose veins, but can also bring about ulcers in the legs through the slow circulation of blood (see Varicose Veins). In this case, the tissues break down to form large, shallow ulcers over the inside of the lower leg and ankle. The ulcers are not particularly painful but may ache considerably.

The immediate treatment for leg ulcers is aimed at keeping the area as free from infection as possible. This includes frequent cleaning, the use of antiseptic ointments or soaks, the application of a sterile foam pad, and firm bandaging (see Dressings and Bandages). Painkilling drugs may also be prescribed. Long-term treatment is also necessary to tackle the underlying cause. This may range from antibiotic therapy to surgery in order to remove or to seal off the defective veins.

Peptic ulcers

The term "peptic" refers to ulcers of the lining of the stomach and of the first part of the small intestine, called the duodenum. These are known, respectively, as gastric and duodenal ulcers, the latter being the more common. Peptic ulceration also includes ulcers forming at the lower end of the esophagus (gullet). The whole of the intestine is lined with a wet membrane called a mucous membrane, and peptic ulcers involve local loss of this membrane, with some penetration into the underlying muscular layer of the big intestine (see Membranes; Mucus). The condition is common, affecting about 10 percent of all adult males and 2 to 5 percent of women. Cigarette smoking interferes with the healing of ulcers and contributes to their causation (see Smoking).

Some of the cells of the stomach lining secrete a powerful hydrochloric acid. This is necessary to help break down food as a preliminary to digestion and to activate an enzyme called pepsin that digests proteins (see Enzymes). Ulcers result when the mechanisms that protect the stomach lining from its own juices have become ineffective and when stomach acid is ejected into the duodenum. In effect, a peptic ulcer is a local partial digestion of the inside of the intestine wall. Normally this does not occur, because the acid and pepsin are present in insufficient quantity and because the linings are protected by mucus and by neutralizing bicarbonate of soda that is secreted by the lining cells.

Various factors interfere with the ability of the lining to resist digestion. These include the taking of certain drugs, especially aspirin and alcohol (see Side Effects), the reflux of bile, and secretions from the duodenum into the stomach. In recent years it has become apparent that the germ *Helicobacter pylori* is also important in bringing about peptic ulceration. Severe head injury, burns, major surgery, and severe infections can also promote peptic ulcers. Ulceration of the lower esophagus occurs when there is considerable upward reflux of acid and pepsin from the stomach (see Esophagus).

Duodenal ulcers

The duodenum is the C-shaped first part of the small intestine. The name comes from its dimensions, said to be equal to the width of 12 fingers. Because the stomach contents empty directly into the duodenum, the first inch or so takes the brunt of this highly irritating mixture, and it is here that duodenal ulcers occur. However, the acid is quickly neutralized by the alkaline digestive juices secreted by the pancreas, the duct of which enters the duodenum at about its midpoint (see Pancreas and Disorders). Duodenal ulcers are local areas in which the intestine wall is being digested by the acid and the pepsin. They do not occur in people who do not secrete stomach acid.

Duodenal ulcers are usually single, but two or more may occur simultaneously. Those that occur on areas of the intestine wall in contact are called kissing ulcers. They are usually about half an inch in diameter (1.3 cm) and penetrate the mucous membrane to erode the muscular coat immediately under the lining. In severe cases, both gastric and duodenal ulcers may pass right through. These are called perforating ulcers and they leave a hole through which the contents of the intestine can escape into the sterile peritoneal cavity of the abdomen surrounding the intestine. This causes a serious

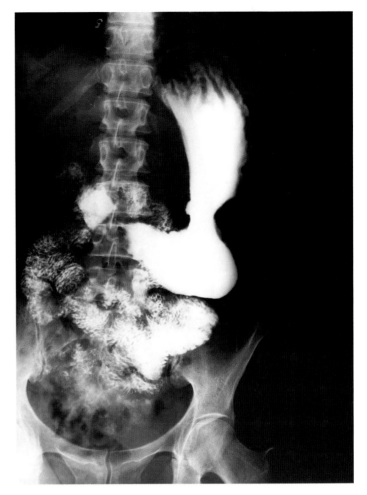

▲ *This X ray shows a gastric ulcer—the small white bulge on the left side of the large white mass (the stomach) to the right of the spinal cord.*

condition, peritonitis (see Peritoneum). Another serious complication of peptic ulceration is severe bleeding caused by the digestion of an artery in the wall of the intestine.

As in gastric ulceration, causal factors of duodenal ulceration include the amount of acid secreted, the efficiency of the mucus secreted by the lining in protecting its own surface from digestion, and the presence of *Helicobacter pylori*. To what extent, and by what means, these and other factors are influenced by the psychological or emotional state of the affected person, or by stress, is not entirely clear, but it is common experience that some forms of stress make symptoms worse (see Stress).

Symptoms of peptic ulcers

Peptic ulceration causes a burning, gnawing pain high in the abdomen in the angle between the ribs. The pain usually comes on about two hours after a meal.

Duodenal ulcer pain is characteristically relieved by taking a small amount of food. This causes the stomach outlet to close, temporarily, so that the new food can be retained for digestion. The pain is not present on waking but tends to come on around the middle of the morning. It is also common for duodenal ulcer pain to wake the sufferer two or three hours after falling asleep. The diagnosis is often apparent from the history but may be confirmed

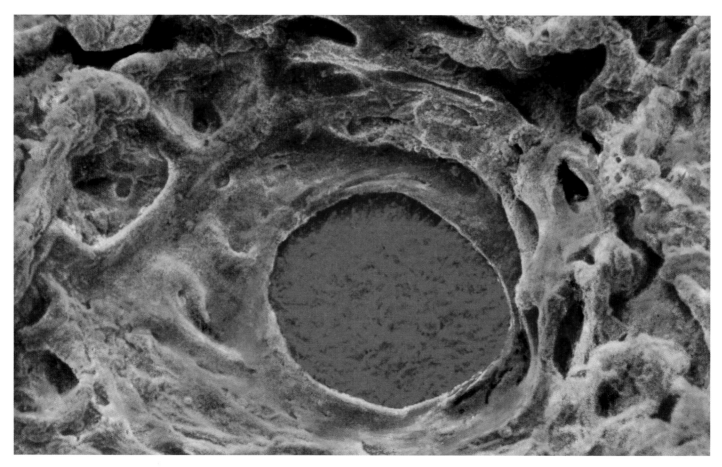

▲ *A micrograph of a gastric ulcer. The round, granular wound is surrounded by a smooth border of cells—the body's attempt to repair the injury—and then the rough texture of healthy gastric mucosa.*

by barium meal X-ray or by direct examination through a flexible illuminating and viewing tube (see Barium Liquids; Endoscopy). Most gastric and duodenal ulcers heal in four to six weeks.

Treatment of peptic ulcer

A wide range of treatments are used. Antibiotics are used to eradicate *Helicobacter pylori* organisms, and bismuth antacid drugs to neutralize stomach acid (see Antibiotics). Histamine H-2 blockers are used to reduce acid secretion, whereas proton pump inhibitor drugs such as omeprazole (Losec) interfere directly with the chemical mechanism by which the acid is formed. Other drugs are used to form a protective coating on the base of the ulcer and promote healing. Prostaglandin drugs are also used, since they have a wide range of actions on cells, some of which can be exploited to cut acid secretion (see Prostaglandins).

In some cases, surgical treatment, such as bypassing the duodenum (gastroenterostomy), reshaping the stomach outlet (pyloroplasty), removing an affected part of the stomach (partial gastrectomy), or cutting some of the nerves to the stomach that promote acid secretion (selective or truncal vagotomy) may be helpful. In addition, treatment with tranquilizing drugs may help by relieving anxiety or depression (see Anxiety; Depression; Tranquilizers).

In spite of treatment, chronic peptic ulceration often persists for life, with relapses every two years or so. The condition is virtually prevented if *Helicobacter pylori* organisms are eliminated. In all cases the outlook will be greatly improved if the patient quits smoking, stops taking aspirin, drinks alcohol only in moderation and in reasonable dilution (see Alcoholism), and reduces dietary intake. Strict diets are not needed; patients need only avoid items known to cause symptoms.

Other ulcers

Pressure sores (which are known medically as decubitus ulcers) commonly affect older, bedridden, and long-term patients. These are caused by constant pressure that impairs the blood circulation through an area of skin and underlying tissue, and commonly occur on the hips, heels, and base of the spine.

The rodent ulcer is a particularly nasty ulcer that occurs on the face. This is actually a type of skin cancer, starting as a red lump that grows and breaks down to form a circular ulcer. Without treatment this continues to grow and spread, but surgical removal or radiation therapy can result in a complete cure. Ulcers can occur in the groin region for many reasons, including sexually acquired herpes or syphilis (see Sexually Transmitted Diseases). Any groin ulcer should be investigated immediately by a doctor, as there is a chance that it may be due to syphilis, which is a very serious disease if it is left untreated.

Any persistent, suspicious, or spreading ulcer should always be taken seriously and brought to the attention of a doctor.

See also: **Bedsores; Colon and colitis; Duodenum; Herpes; Mouth; Skin and skin diseases; Sores; Stomach; Syphilis; Vagotomy**

Ultrasound

Questions and Answers

Our doctor says that my father needs ultrasound treatment for his shoulder, which is stiff and painful. Will he have to have a scan?

No. Ultrasound has many other uses in medicine besides scanning. In physical therapy, ultrasound beams provide deep heat and promote healing of inflamed tissues, especially around joints.

When my pregnant wife had an ultrasound scan, the doctor told her to drink plenty of water one hour in advance. Why?

Ultrasound examinations in pregnancy are always performed with the bladder as full as possible because this lifts the uterus into the correct position for a scan and pushes other organs out of the way. In addition, the urine in the bladder transmits ultrasound well, and greatly improves the quality of the image attained.

Is it easy to tell the gender of a fetus by ultrasound scanning?

Yes, modern high-resolution ultrasound machines can readily show up the sex of the fetus toward the end of pregnancy. Most obstetricians or ultrasound technicians will inquire whether you want to know.

My friend had a kidney transplant last year and has had a number of ultrasound scans. What could all of these scans show?

Ultrasonography is a good way to follow the progress of transplant patients because it is harmless and gives a clear view of the transplant. Two important complications can be detected with ultrasound: any rejection or any obstruction of the kidney. Without ultrasound, frequent X-ray examinations would have to be made; these carry a much greater risk.

One of modern medicine's significant advances is the use of very high-frequency sound to investigate the interior of the body. Ultrasound has added a wonderfully effective weapon to the doctor's diagnostic armory.

Sound reflection technology is not new. Over 80 years ago it was used to probe the North Atlantic in the hunt for the wreck of the *Titanic*. Over 50 years ago its use in sonar equipment was of strategic importance during World War II. Ultrasound technology is now used in most branches of industry and science, and its impact on medical diagnosis has been far-reaching, especially in obstetrics, where its safety and the information it provides about the fetus have made great advances possible (see Fetus; Obstetrics).

How ultrasound works

The higher the frequency of sound, the shorter the wavelength. If sound is to be reflected from small areas, it must be of very short wavelengths. Audible sound requires areas like mountains or the seabed to reflect it and produce echoes. For medical purposes, frequencies of many millions of cycles per second (megahertz) are required to produce wavelengths short enough to be reflected from internal body surfaces. Such frequencies are easily produced by electronic oscillators and the sound waves are produced by piezoelectric crystals in a handheld device called a transducer, or probe, that both emits the waves and detects the echoes.

The transducer produces 20 or more pulses of ultrasound per second, and each pulse is so brief in duration, lasting a mere millionth of a second, that there is a relatively long interval between pulses. During these intervals, the probe picks up any echoes reflected from the tissues within the body. Analysis of the echo pattern is a complex process that requires a computer, but the final result is usually an image on a monitor screen that represents a cross section or slice through the body along the path of the probe.

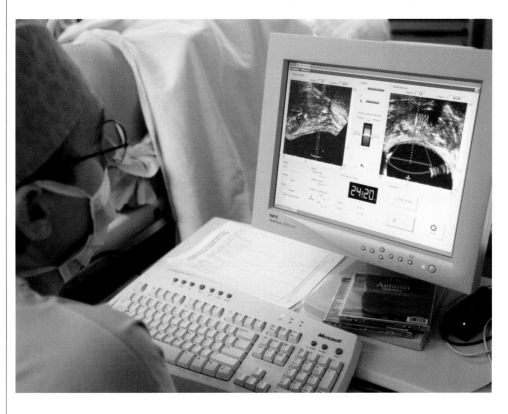

▲ *A doctor studies an ultrasound scan of a patient suspected of having prostate cancer.*

Questions and Answers

This is my first pregnancy, and my baby is due in four weeks' time. I have now had five ultrasound scans because the obstetrician was worried about the position of the placenta. Now he says that everything is fine, but I am terribly worried that so many scans may have harmed the baby in some way. Could anything have happened?

Doctors have enormous experience with ultrasound in pregnancy, and careful research all over the world has failed to show any evidence of harmful effects. The possible risks and benefits of every procedure used in medicine require consideration. In your case, the risk was negligible, and the benefit great. So, don't worry at all.

My wife is now 28 weeks pregnant, and so far all seems well. However, shouldn't she have had an ultrasound scan to make sure that everything is all right with the baby?

Yes. Modern ultrasound provides so much valuable information about the state of the fetus and the progress of the pregnancy that in the Western world it is now considered almost routine for every pregnant woman to have an ultrasound scan. Current prenatal tests of fetal well-being are principally based on ultrasound examinations and can identify those fetuses in the early stages of asphyxia. Doppler ultrasound can provide continuous records of the fetal heart rate. Your wife is most certainly scheduled for ultrasound examination.

Last time my sister-in-law went to the prenatal clinic, the doctor used a special instrument to let her hear the baby's heartbeat. Was this an ultrasound machine?

Yes, it was. Blood flowing through the fetal heart reflects ultrasound in a characteristic way; and numerous devices are available that process echoes returning from the heart into an audible sound, usually a loud whooshing noise.

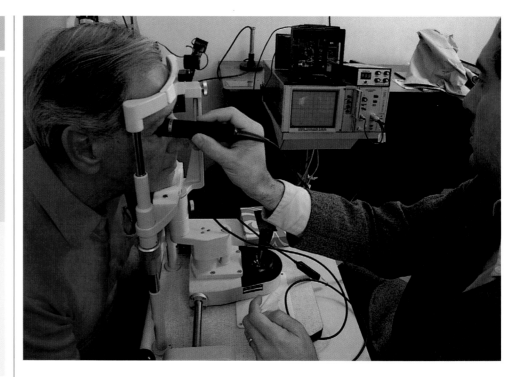

▲ *This patient is undergoing an ultrasound examination of the eye. The probe emits high-frequency sound waves and is held by a technician, while an image is built up on the monitor screen in the background.*

One further property of ultrasound is of great importance: ultrasound is not a form of nuclear radiation and does not affect living tissues in the way that such radiation does. It is almost certainly harmless. This is one major advantage that ultrasound has over X rays.

Having an ultrasound scan

An ultrasound scan is an entirely painless procedure performed by a doctor or technician with special training. After an initial explanation, the patient is asked to undress to expose the region to be examined. He or she then lies down on a couch. A thin layer of oil or gel is applied to the skin to facilitate contact with the probe and improve the quality of the image. The lights are dimmed during the procedure so that the image on the screen may be viewed to best advantage and the probe is passed gently to and fro over the area under examination.

There is no special preparation needed for an ultrasound scan and the patient to be scanned does not need to stay in the hospital either before or after the procedure unless the scan reveals something that needs treatment.

Different types of ultrasound equipment produce different types of images, such as moving pictures or a sequence of still pictures, both of which can be recorded for further analysis and review.

Ultrasound in pregnancy

Perhaps the most important use of the ultrasound technique is in pregnancy. Here it yields a wealth of information about the fetus, at an important early stage and with no risk to the fetus or the mother. The information gained can have a crucial bearing upon the outcome of the pregnancy for mother and fetus that is not easily obtained by any other method of examination.

Ultrasonography is used to detect multiple pregnancies, and to determine the position of the fetus and precise location of the placenta. It may be used to screen for fetal abnormalities such as spina bifida, and it also assists with the detection of other problems when used as a guide in amniocentesis (see Spina Bifida).

Accurate measurements of the fetus may be taken throughout pregnancy and are used to monitor fetal growth or to predict the date of delivery. Even the beating heart of the fetus can be detected by ultrasound, giving rapid and efficient confirmation that all is well. X rays are still needed during pregnancy in certain circumstances, usually in situations when accurate measurement of the mother's pelvis becomes necessary (see X Rays).

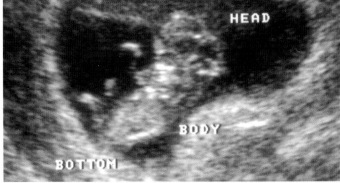

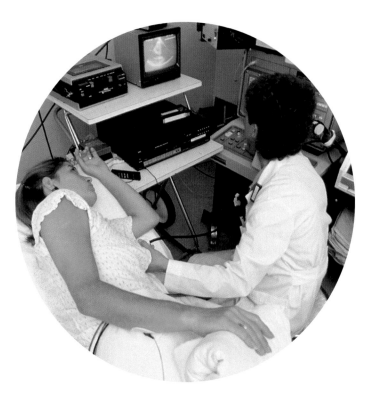

▲ *This young woman is undergoing an ultrasound scan, or echocardiography. The scan gives a clear picture of the patient's heart, which is reflected as an image on the monitor screen in the background.*

The development of many ultrasound techniques and their increasingly widespread availability have brought about a revolution in obstetric care that removes much of the guesswork, thereby making both pregnancy and childbirth much safer.

Diagnosis

Ultrasound is also used to investigate and diagnose diseases that change either the shape or the sound-reflecting properties of organs accessible to the ultrasound beam. Air, bone, and fat interfere with the ability of ultrasound to form satisfactory images that can be seen on the screen, since ultrasound waves cannot pass through bone or gas. Organs such as the lungs, the intestines, and the brain are unsuitable for examination.

Ultrasound pictures of the heart have brought about almost as great a revolution as those of the growing fetus. For an ultrasound scan of the heart, a probe is pointed between the ribs and excellent pictures of the movement of heart valves and of the chambers of the heart can be obtained (see Heart). This is especially useful in the investigation of heart problems in children, and progress is being made in diagnosing the heart problems of babies in the womb.

The abdomen, liver, gallbladder, spleen, pancreas, and kidneys can be seen clearly on an ultrasound scan. Cysts, tumors, abscesses, and stones, together with many other types of abnormality, can also be detected in these organs by means of ultrasonography. Obstruction in the bile duct or in the kidneys can be shown, and ultrasound also provides valuable information about the extent of cancer spread (see Bile; Cancer; Kidneys and Kidney Diseases). The major blood vessels in the abdomen are very easily identified, and abnormalities can be detected by the technique.

▲▼ *The ultrasound scan above shows a fetus in the womb at 12 weeks. The scan below is the fetus at 20 weeks, and it is easy to see that baby's head and arms are more clearly defined and developed. Ultrasonography reveals to the obstetrician a great deal of vital information about the growth of the fetus.*

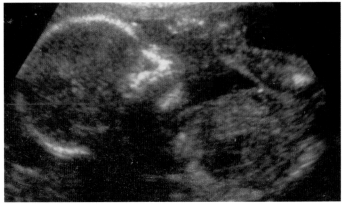

Ultrasound can also be used for difficult biopsy procedures, thereby reducing the hazard to the patient (see Biopsy).

Another useful application for ultrasound is its ability to distinguish between cysts and tumors in the thyroid gland, the breast, and ovarian tissue. It is sometimes even used in diagnosing disease of the prostate gland. In the eye, ultrasound can be used to diagnose common problems such as a detached retina, and to locate foreign bodies within the eyeball following injury.

Outlook

The technique of ultrasonography is still under development and more applications are being constantly considered. Techniques now being developed include the use of ultrasound to make precise measurements of bodily functions, such as rates of blood flow to different organs. A newer application of the technique is to use it to treat soft-tissue injuries.

Intensive research in ultrasound technology continues to gain momentum, and many people will benefit from its results over the decades to come. The ability to see inside the body without causing any disturbance or harm will continue to be of extreme importance in the constant battle against disease and illness.

See also: **Amniocentesis; Diagnostic imaging; Heat treatment; Physical therapy; Pregnancy; Prenatal care; Scans**

Unconsciousness

While playing football, I was kicked on the head and lost consciousness. I was kept in the hospital overnight and told that for a time I should not read or go back to work if I had to concentrate hard. Why was this?

Concussion has degrees of severity, and, although a patient may feel fit, the effects can last for up to two weeks. A person who has suffered a concussion may have recurrent headaches and nausea, but these symptoms will disappear. However, it has been found that reading, bright lights, and deep concentration can delay recovery.

What is the difference between fainting and being unconscious?

Fainting is a very light form of unconsciousness caused by a lack of oxygen reaching the brain. The person quickly recovers when blood circulation is restored. A person who is unconscious cannot be easily roused, and may show confusion, forgetfulness, and even stupor when he or she finally comes around. The condition is more serious than a simple faint: it can be brought on by a variety of causes that threaten health.

If I get knocked out when boxing, will my brain be damaged?

A knockout implies significant brain damage but usually recovery appears to be full. There may be bruising of the brain and small hemorrhages in the tissues. If you have had a number of knockouts, or you lose consciousness easily, you must be examined by a doctor. There may be damage from an earlier concussion. There is no treatment and you should not continue to box. The effects of brain damage may not be obvious. Many boxers who show few obvious effects have suffered permanent damage.

Slipping into unconsciousness can be dangerous. Brought on by a variety of causes, unconsciousness can range in severity from a fleeting faint to a life-threatening or permanent coma.

Normal consciousness may be defined as a state in which a person is awake, alert, and aware of his or her environment. Unconsciousness is a sleeplike state, but much deeper, with the person having no awareness of the surroundings and showing no response to any stimuli. It can vary in severity, ranging from a transient faint to a prolonged coma. Whatever its immediate cause, the condition arises because of important changes in the brain (see Brain).

Mechanisms in the brain

Exactly how the brain functions in consciousness and unconsciousness is not yet fully understood. However, there are a number of critical areas in the brain that are deeply involved in maintaining consciousness. These are the cerebral cortex, the thalamus, the brain stem, and, in particular, a group of cells within the brain stem called the reticular formation.

The cerebral cortex receives sensory inputs from the main sensory nerves and also from the reticular formation. Nerve routes from around the body branch out to the reticular formation and feed it a constant stream of electrical signals. This action, in turn, causes the reticular formation to fire off signals to targets all around the brain, to the appropriate centers that gather, collate, and act upon the signals. If this driving force slows down, or is prevented from occurring, the cerebral cortex becomes sleepy, and as a result we become unconscious. The brain stem is also important in that it is responsible for keeping essential body mechanisms, such as heartbeat, blood pressure, and breathing, running smoothly without a person's consciously

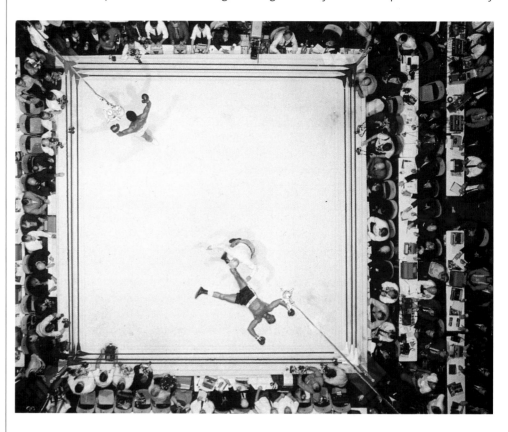

▲ *Cleveland Williams lies prostrate in the ring after being knocked unconscious by Mohammed Ali in Houston, Texas, in 1966.*

having to think about them. It appears that when someone becomes unconscious, for whatever reason, the brain concentrates on keeping the body ticking over by using all available energy to maintain normal brain stem function. Damage is thereby confined to nonessential areas of the brain.

Degrees of unconsciousness

The activity of the brain is measured by electroencephalography (EEG). The impulses of the brain are presented as a pattern of electrical waves, which varies according to the degree of alertness or unconsciousness, thus providing a clue to the severity of the unconscious state. For instance, during unconsciousness, the pattern of waves is slow and large, usually about three waves each second. If someone is coming around from unconsciousness or waking from sleep, the waves come at about six to eight a second and increase in frequency until, at full consciousness, the pattern of waves is rapid and jagged, showing increased electrical activity. The EEG machine is used to determine whether the brain has been severely damaged or even died. If the EEG shows no electrical

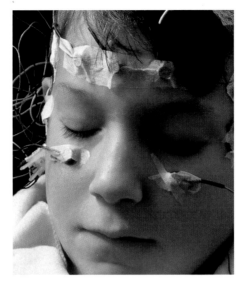

◄ A boy having electroencephalography (EEG). Electrodes are attached to the head and face to record electrical activity in different areas of the brain. This is used to form a multichannel tracing of brain electrical activity that can be compared with a normal control subject.

activity, then the person has almost certainly suffered brain death.

Unconsciousness can be caused by a variety of factors, ranging from shock to poisoning. The most likely cause is syncope, or fainting (see Fainting). Fainting can be brought on by excessive heat or by standing still for long periods, conditions that result in a temporary lack of blood supply to the brain. The resultant lack of oxygen forces the brain to shut down for a short time until the oxygen supply is restored to normal levels. If, for some reason, the blood supply to the brain is not fully and quickly restored the person may enter a deeper state of unconsciousness.

Symptoms of fainting include dizziness (see Dizziness), light-headedness, and pallor of the face. Someone who has fainted should lie down for a few minutes until a full recovery has been made. Allowing people who have fainted to get up too soon, or pulling them to their feet, could result in a more serious unconscious state.

Poisoning due to fumes, chemicals, or drugs can cause unconsciousness, though by a different mechanism. For instance, barbiturates depress the central nervous system, in which case the brain stem may be affected, necessitating emergency measures to ensure the maintenance of the life-support systems. Stimulants will

▼ The sound of the alarm enters the brain through the ear, but the sleeper reacts only when the reticular formation awakens the brain by sending signals to the appropriate area of the cerebral cortex. If someone is unconscious, for whatever reason, the reticular formation is not functioning, so although sensory information arrives at the cortex the person remains unaware of it.

SLEEP VERSUS UNCONSCIOUSNESS

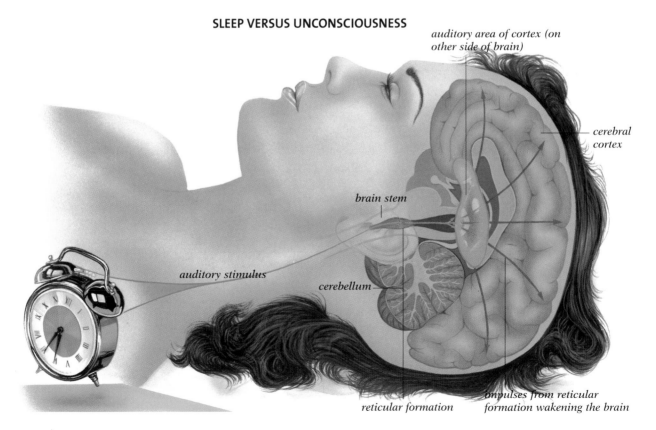

auditory area of cortex (on other side of brain)

cerebral cortex

brain stem

auditory stimulus

cerebellum

reticular formation

impulses from reticular formation wakening the brain

Questions and Answers

My young daughter often gets into a rage and then faints. Could she be epileptic?

If you suspect that your daughter is suffering from epilepsy, you should consult your doctor as soon as possible. What you describe could be a condition known as breath-holding. This can resemble an epileptic attack but it usually occurs only in children of between one and four years of age and during a severe temper or crying fit. Usually they let out a cry before turning blue in the face and passing out. There may be small convulsions. Although these attacks can be frightening for parents, they are not serious, and a child will grow out of them. But it is important to have the condition properly diagnosed.

Why do pilots ejecting from a plane sometimes black out?

This kind of blackout generally occurs when there is rapid acceleration of the body and blood is suddenly drained away from the head. Momentary unconsciousness occurs as the brain is briefly starved of oxygen.

A friend of mine did not become unconscious when hit on the head, but lapsed into unconsciousness later. Why?

This emphasizes the serious nature of any blow on the head. Even a minor blow can have a serious, delayed effect in that unconsciousness can follow some time later. This may often be preceded by vomiting and violent headaches, and indicates that there is a high probability that slow bleeding is occurring within the skull, usually external to the brain. Because the adult skull cannot expand, such bleeding compresses the brain and pushes it downward to the opening for the spinal cord, thereby compressing the vital centers in the brain stem. Unless stopped, it is invariably fatal. Such a situation calls for immediate emergency neurosurgical intervention if life is to be saved.

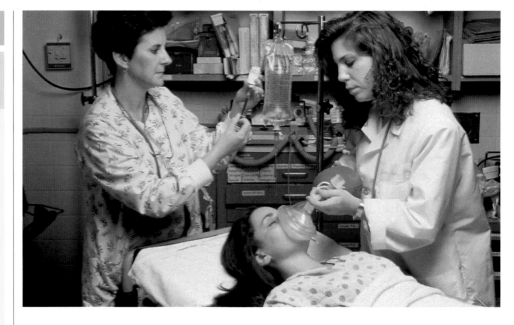

▲ *An unconscious woman is given oxygen in the hospital emergency department.*

be given to treat this type of poisoning when it has led to an unconscious state. Carbon monoxide poisoning, however, replaces oxygen in the blood and leads to an oxygen deficiency in the brain. To treat this, the person must be removed immediately from the source of the gas and given artificial respiration (see Poisoning).

Shock can bring on unconsciousness owing to a collapse of the circulatory system. Once the circulatory system fails to maintain an adequate supply of blood to the brain, the collection of symptoms known as shock syndrome becomes apparent. This includes sweating, blurred vision, shallow, rapid breathing, and faintness that can result in unconsciousness.

Shock can also be brought on by extensive internal or external bleeding, heart attacks, and loss of body fluid due to various illnesses. For example, in cholera, the body becomes so dehydrated

▼ *A doctor prepares a patient for an EEG. The procedure is a useful diagnostic tool. Waveforms indicate conditions such as epilepsy, dementia, and drug disturbances.*

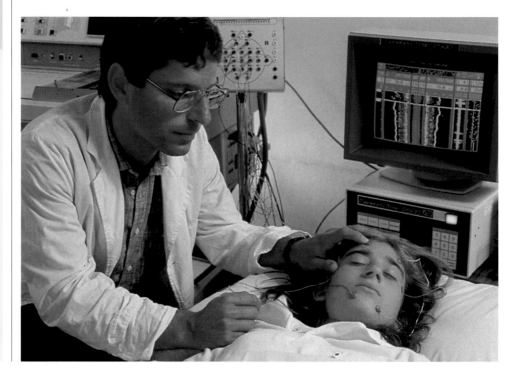

Some common causes of unconsciousness

TYPE	CAUSE	ACTION
Fainting (syncope)	Lack of blood supplying the brain	Lie the patient flat. Cold water or smelling salts may help.
Concussion	Blow to the head. Blood vessels contract and starve the brain of blood.	Keep patient in quiet and darkened room until he or she comes around. Up to two weeks in bed. No stimulant drugs at all but maybe painkillers to ease headache. Visit doctor's office for checkup.
Electric shock	Faulty wiring, lightning. Paralysis of breathing centers in brain.	Turn off the power source. Give mouth-to-mouth resuscitation and heart massage, if necessary. Keep it up until medical help arrives.
Stroke	Collapse of blood vessel in the brain or blockage by blood clot	Call paramedics immediately. Leave victim alone but place something under his or her head.
Poisoning	A variety of poisons have a number of effects	Call doctor. Give mouth-to-mouth resuscitation if the victim is not breathing; if poison is in mouth give mouth-to-nose. If victim is breathing, place in the recovery position. Do not leave victim alone.
Infections such as malaria, cholera, and meningitis	Invading organisms	The illness must be treated by a doctor. When a patient slips into unconsciousness, make sure he or she can breathe easily; then inform the doctor immediately.
Hypoglycemia	Too much insulin or too little carbohydrate	Give sugar drink or glucagon injection and call paramedics.
Diabetic coma	Too little insulin or too much carbohydrate in the diet	Call doctor to give insulin and sugar.
Epilepsy	Cause unknown but spontaneous dysfunction of the brain	Lie the victim down away from anything that may cause injury. Turn him or her on one side and make sure air passages are clear. Place rolled-up handkerchief, or something similar, between the teeth if possible. This prevents tongue biting. Call paramedics.
Shock	Severe bleeding Allergic shock reaction to injection Rarely, bee stings Internal injuries Heart and circulatory problems	Call paramedics. Stop bleeding if possible. Keep victim cool. Reassure and keep him or her calm.

that the sufferer dies of shock rather than of the bacterium. The treatment of shock depends on its cause. Replacing lost fluid and raising the blood pressure are measures taken in the hospital, but it is important to stop heavy bleeding as soon as possible. If patients become unconscious, they should be turned to one side to ensure that they can breathe properly. If breathing stops, artificial respiration must be given (see Shock).

Head injuries that occur in sports are a common cause of unconsciousness, which may be caused by direct injury to brain tissue or by a temporary contraction of blood vessels that impairs brain function. This condition is known as concussion, and varies in severity. A return to consciousness may be accompanied by headache, nausea, and difficulty focusing. Loss of memory of events that happened before the injury is a symptom of concussion. Anyone who has been knocked out should see a doctor as soon as possible, since there may be damage to the skull or internal bleeding.

Epilepsy can also lead to unconsciousness and is usually accompanied by convulsions of differing severity. It is not known why the fit occurs but it is brought on by an uncontrollable discharge of electricity by the brain (see Epilepsy).

Coma

A coma is the most extreme form of unconsciousness. It is serious and often long-lasting. The activity of the brain is depressed, and even reflex actions such as coughing, corneal reflexes, and tendon reflexes are absent. In the very deepest coma, the person may not respond even to a painful stimuli (see Coma). The usual causes of coma are injury to the brain (such as bleeding or tumor), severe shock, and blood poisoning. Damage to the thalamus may initiate a permanent coma. Diabetes and hypoglycemia are also common causes of a coma, but these conditions can be controlled.

In the past, any kind of coma that lasted for more than 24 hours usually resulted in permanent brain damage, but modern treatment and nursing have done much to change this. However, the longer a coma lasts, the less likelihood there is that a perfect recovery can be made. In all cases of unconsciousness, treatment depends on the underlying cause, and may range from simple rest and recuperation to surgery. A comatose patient will require long-term care.

See also: **Barbiturates; Diabetes; Hypoglycemia**

Uremia

Questions and Answers

Uremia is a condition that generally, but not always, develops as a result of kidney malfunction. Treatment through dialysis or kidney transplant is strikingly effective for most patients.

If uremia is diagnosed, will the patient have to be put on a kidney machine or have a transplant?

Anyone with a high level of breakdown products, such as urea, in the blood, is said to be uremic. There may be several causes, but one of the most common is that the kidneys can no longer cope with the demands made on them. This condition is called chronic renal failure. In these circumstances, an alternative method of clearing waste products from the blood will have to be used. A transplant or some form of dialysis is the usual treatment.

My grandfather went into the hospital to have prostate surgery and the doctors discovered that he was uremic. Is this common?

Elderly patients often suffer from prostate difficulties, which obstruct the flow of urine from the bladder. If this persists, pressure builds up on the kidneys, leading to uremia.

Can diet help to control uremia?

Yes. Before substitutes for kidney function were developed, dietary restrictions were used to prolong the lives of people with chronic renal failure. Excessive urea accumulates from deficient metabolism of protein by the kidneys, so the basis of all dietary treatment for uremia is to reduce the amount of protein.

Does uremia inevitably lead to serious kidney trouble?

No. Elderly patients often have a raised level of urea in the blood without serious consequences, simply because their kidneys are older and working less efficiently. Dehydration can also produce high levels of urea in fit people, but this form of uremia will respond simply to taking in a lot of liquid.

Many kidney diseases involve an accumulation of waste products in the body. Urea is the major waste product and a high level causes uremia to develop.

Causes

The kidney's main function is to filter urea, creatinine, and uric acid from the blood (see Excretory Systems). Kidney problems start if between half and three-quarters of the individual kidney tubules or nephrons stop working, leading to a buildup of urea in the blood, and chronic renal failure results.

However, a diseased kidney is not the only cause of uremia. If the blood supply to the kidney is interrupted, urine is no longer produced, owing to shock, and the blood pressure drops for a period of time. This will damage the kidneys and they can take days or even weeks to recover.

Uremia may develop if the flow of urine is impeded, as with an obstruction of the prostate gland in a man (see Prostate Gland).

Symptoms and treatment

Over a long period a patient may develop fairly severe uremia without actually realizing that there is anything seriously wrong. The main symptoms of the disease

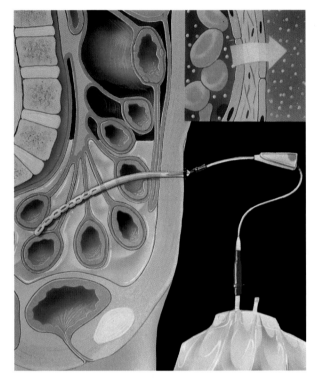

▲ *This illustration of a section through the human abdomen shows the technique of peritoneal dialysis. This is the infusion of dialysis fluid from a plastic bag directly into the peritoneal cavity via a plastic catheter. The process removes waste products from the body fluids of a person whose kidneys do not function properly. The principle of dialysis is that waste products in blood diffuse across a semipermeable membrane, in this case the peritoneal membrane, toward the lower solute concentrations of the dialysis fluid.*

are a general feeling of ill health and lack of energy. Uremia also affects the way that the bone marrow makes blood, and, as a result, anemia may complicate the patient's condition (see Anemia).

The brain may be affected as the uremia worsens: the patient may be sleepy and confused until he or she loses consciousness. The skin is dry and turns sallow. Some of the waste products normally excreted through the kidney are lost in sweat, resulting in severe itching.

When uremia is due to chronic renal failure, treatment is by a kidney transplant or dialysis (see Kidney Transplants). Dialysis uses a machine to remove urea from the blood. Another form of dialysis uses fluid flowing in and out of the peritoneal cavity. Urea passes across the peritoneum from the blood into the fluid, which is then drained (see Peritoneum).

See also: **Blood pressure; Kidney dialysis; Kidneys and kidney diseases; Shock**

Urethra

Questions and Answers

Is urethritis always caused by a sexually transmitted disease?

No, but a sexually transmitted infection is the most common cause. This is because the penis in men and the area around the vagina that includes the opening of the urethra in women are usually in close contact during intercourse. Women may also get urethritis through contamination from the anus; to avoid this, they should always wipe themselves after defecating, or dry themselves after bathing, from the front toward the back, never the opposite.

Can urethritis always be cured?

Yes, almost always, though this depends on doing tests to identify the precise cause so that the appropriate treatment, usually an antibiotic, can be given. However, Just taking the antibiotic may not be enough to produce a cure, since like any other infected area of the body, the urethra needs a period of rest for full recovery. New lining tissue can then become established and replace that which has been destroyed by the inflammation. It is usually necessary to refrain from intercourse for about two weeks or the mechanical stress and friction on the urethra will damage the new lining tissue before it has had a chance to settle down, causing a further attack of urethritis.

A friend told me that her little boy had hypospadias. What is that?

Hypospadias is an abnormality in the development of the penis. This occurs before birth and as a result the opening, or meatus, is on the underside of the penis rather than at the tip. In most cases there is no difficulty in passing urine, having intercourse, or fathering children, and no treatment is necessary. In the few cases where there is a problem, it can be corrected with minor surgery.

The urethra is a channel from the bladder to an opening on the outside of the body along which urine is discharged. It is a common site of urethritis—an infection that can be very painful and always needs medical attention.

CROSS SECTION OF THE URETHRA

The male and female urethras. Notice the proximity of the bladder to the urethral opening in each; in the female the urethra is much shorter and therefore more exposed to infection.

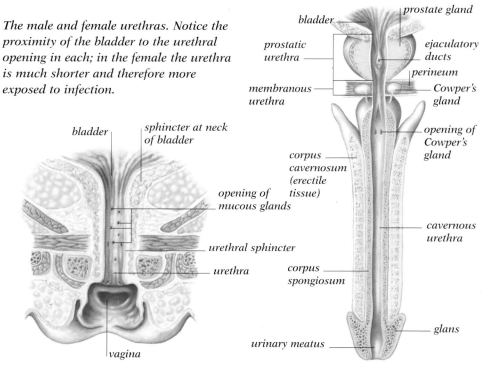

The mature male urethra averages 8 inches (about 20 cm) in length and consists of three sections. The first, or prostatic, section is about 1 inch (2.5 cm) long and passes from the sphincter, or valve, at the outlet of the bladder through the middle of the prostate gland. The middle part of the urethra is only about 0.5 inch (12 mm) long and is often called the membranous urethra. The final—and, at over 6 inches (15 cm), the longest—section is called the spongy or cavernous urethra. This section is within the penis and opens at the slit in the tip, the urethral meatus. In men, the urethra is also the channel through which semen is ejaculated (see Erection and Ejaculation).

In women the only function of the urethra is as a channel for urine disposal. Surrounded by mucous glands, it is much shorter—about 1.5 inches (4 cm) in length. Because of its shortness, and because it opens into a relatively exposed, contaminated area, women often get urinary infections.

Urethritis

Inflammation of the urethra (see Inflammation), called urethritis, is the most common urethral disorder. It can have many causes, the most common of which is sexual intercourse with an infected partner. The symptoms in the male are a discharge that leaks out from the urethral meatus, increasing pain on urinating, and a desire to urinate frequently. In women, usually only the pain (dysuria) and the frequency of urination are present. These symptoms are often attributed to cystitis or inflammation of the bladder, but it is more commonly the urethra that is involved. If urethritis is not fully treated, usually with antibiotics, permanent damage can be done both to the urethra itself and to the reproductive organs (see Antibiotics).

See also: **Bladder and bladder problems; Cystitis; Penis and disorders; Prostate gland; Semen; Sexually transmitted diseases**

Urinary tract and disorders

My son, who is seven, has urinary tract problems. A urologist arranged for him to have an X-ray while he was urinating. Is this a proper kind of test?

Yes. It is used extensively in children. It is called micturating cystourethrography (MCU), which just means an X-ray of the bladder and the outlet tube (the urethra) while the patient is urinating. It is useful in investigating abnormal bladder emptying and abnormalities in the urethra.

Is it true that women are more prone to cystitis than men? And if so, why is this?

Urinary tract infections are more common in women than in men. This is generally thought to be because the urethra is much shorter in women than in men and its external opening is more easily contaminated than a man's. The idea is encouraged by the fact that most urinary infections in women are due to coliform organisms. This is not the whole story; the symptoms of cystitis, in the absence of any infection, are also more common in women than in men.

My mother is 70 and often has urinary infections. She needs to go to the toilet several times during the night but produces only a small amount of urine. Last week I persuaded her to see the doctor and he prescribed an estrogen vaginal cream. Why?

Many cases of postmenopausal urinary infection are the direct result of an atrophic condition of the vagina from estrogen deficiency. This leads to a change in normal healthy vaginal bacteria and frequent bladder infections. There's a good chance that this prescription will clear up your mother's problems.

The urinary tract is one of the major systems of the body. It has the important function of disposing of waste products that would, if retained, eventually cause serious illness or death. The urinary tract system is prone to a wide range of disorders.

The urinary tract consists of two kidneys; two tubes called ureters that run down from the kidneys to enter the back of the base of the bladder; the expansible muscular bladder itself with its control sphincter; and a single outlet tube, the urethra, that carries urine from the bladder to the exterior. In women, the reproductive system is entirely separate from the urinary tract, but in men, these functions are partly combined and the urethra is a conduit for seminal fluid as well as urine. Another important difference between the sexes is that in males the part of the urethra immediately below the bladder is surrounded by a gland, the prostate gland, that tends, in elderly men, to enlarge and obstruct the outflow of urine.

Function of the urinary tract

The kidneys have several vital functions. They regulate the total volume of fluid in the body and the chemical composition of that fluid. They remove the waste material produced by the body's metabolic processes, mainly urea from protein breakdown, uric acid from DNA and RNA, creatinine from muscle, and bilirubin from red blood cells. The kidneys excrete drugs. They can synthesize glucose during starvation; they also secrete hormones that promote new blood cell formation, control blood pressure, and influence calcium balance.

Urine produced by the kidneys, at an average rate of about 1 ml per minute, passes down the ureters to be stored in the bladder. This is an unconscious process for a time because the bladder expands easily as it fills. The adult bladder has a capacity of 12–15 fluid ounces (350–450 ml), but can expand to about 24 fluid ounces (700 ml) if urination is deliberately delayed. At that point of expansion, however, voluntary control is lost.

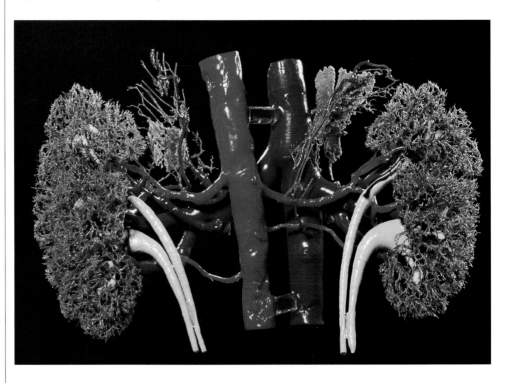

▲ *A resin corrosion cast shows the blood vessels of the kidneys. The arteries are red, the veins are blue, and the ureters and renal pelvis are yellow.*

Nephritis

The most common form of kidney inflammation affecting the urine-producing parts of the organ is called glomerulonephritis. This is not the result of an infection but is caused by abnormal functioning of the immune system (autoimmune disease) following the production of antibodies to a streptococcal infection (see Immune System). Most cases cause no serious long-term effects, but a small proportion proceed to a long-term or chronic state that may end in total loss of kidney function, that is, kidney failure. This will require dialysis or kidney transplantation (see Kidneys and Kidney Diseases). Nephrosis is a chronic degenerative disease of the kidney substance, and there is severe loss of protein in the urine. It may follow glomerulonephritis, other diseases, or drug reactions.

Urinary tract infections

Like every other system in the body, the urinary tract is subject to a wide range of diseases and disorders. The most common of these are infections. Urethritis is inflammation of the lining of the urethra, usually from sexually acquired infection. The common causes are chlamydia and gonococci (see Inflammation).

Infection of the urinary bladder is very common, especially in women; 80 percent of the germs are coliform species from the lower bowel. Many other germs can, however, can infect the bladder. Infection can spread upward from the bladder to the kidneys to cause pyelonephritis: acute or chronic infection of the urine collecting systems (see Bladder and Bladder Problems). Abscesses can occur in the kidney tissue and primary infections of the kidneys with germs such as the tubercle bacillus may occur.

Urinary tract cancer

Cancer of the penis is rare, especially if personal hygiene is good, with daily washing. Apart from prostate cancer, which is one of the most common of all kinds of cancer, bladder cancer is the most frequent form of urinary tract cancer. It accounts for 7 percent of

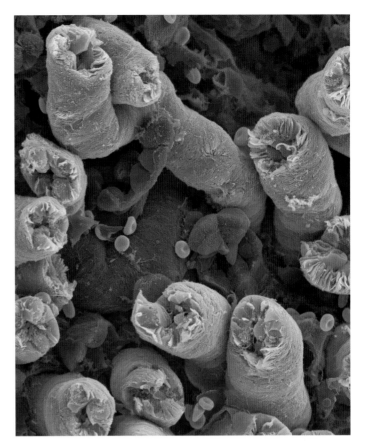

▲ *A scanning electron micrograph of nephrons, the filtration tubules in the kidney, magnified 140 times. Nephrons are the functional units of the kidney; they filter out metabolic waste.*

new cancers in men and 3 percent in women. It is mainly due to cigarette smoking and exposure to industrial carcinogens. Bladder cancer can be diagnosed by direct visual examination through a cystoscope and the taking of biopsy samples. The outlook depends on the stage which the disease has reached at the time of diagnosis.

Cancer of the kidney accounts for about 3 percent of adult cancers. The only consistently linked risk factor is cigarette smoking. Again, the outlook depends on the stage at the time of detection. Wilms' tumor (nephroblastoma) is a rare congenital kidney cancer that shows itself in the first three years of life. Treatment of both bladder and kidney cancers is mainly surgical.

Other urinary tract disorders

Congenital defects of the urinary tract are fairly common. They include absent kidneys, underdeveloped kidneys, joined kidneys (horseshoe kidney), and multicystic kidneys, a condition in which cysts replace normal tissue until the kidneys fail completely. Polycystic kidneys in adults are due to the late effects of congenital defects in the tubular system.

Stone formation is common in the urinary tract and this may occur in the kidneys or in the bladder. Kidney stones passing down the ureters cause severe pain called renal colic. Stones can be broken up by focused sound waves (extracorporeal shock wave lithotripsy).

See also: Infection and infectious diseases

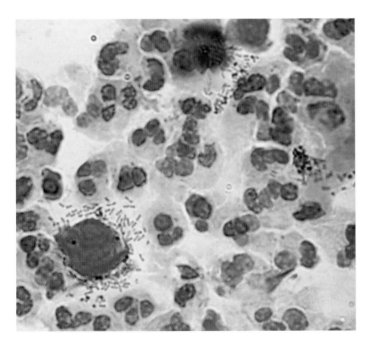

▲ *A gram-stained micrograph of a urethral discharge shows the presence of* Trichomonas vaginalis.

Uterus

Questions and Answers

Does the Pill affect the uterus?

Yes. There are several types of contraceptive pill, all containing a synthetic form of progesterone at levels that make the endometrium, or lining of the uterus, unsuitable for the implantation and growth of a fertilized egg. The Pill affects the secretions from the cervix to prevent sperm from swimming through the cervix to fertilize the egg. Many contraceptive pills also contain a synthetic estrogen. This helps to prevent pregnancy by inhibiting the release of eggs from the ovary.

Is it true that some women may go into premature labor because the cervix is too weak to remain closed until the baby is mature?

Doctors are often unable to tell a woman why she had her baby prematurely, and one preterm birth is a source of anxiety for any subsequent pregnancies. Occasionally a woman has an abnormal cervix that can be stretched open too easily; it can usually be treated by putting a purse-string type of suture into the neck of the womb to keep it closed. This is inserted under anesthesia, and is removed when the woman is in the 38th week of pregnancy.

Why do women stop menstruating at menopause?

When a woman menstruates she sheds the lining to the womb, called the endometrium. The endometrium is stimulated to grow by two ovarian hormones, estrogen and progesterone. At menopause the ovaries no longer secrete the hormones, the endometrium does not regrow, and the woman has no more periods. The onset of menopause is around 45 to 55. If periods are heavier or more frequent during this time, a doctor should be consulted.

The workings of the uterus are something of a medical mystery. What is undeniable, however, is that it is perfectly adapted for the protection and nurturing of an unborn child.

In the past, the uterus has been blamed for almost every mental and physical ailment women suffer. Today we have a more rational, though still incomplete, understanding of this vital organ.

The uterus is composed of two main parts; the corpus or body of the organ, and its cervix or neck (see Cervix and Cervical Smears). It is capable of undergoing major changes during a woman's reproductive life.

From puberty to menopause, the lining of the womb (endometrium) develops each month under the influence of hormones to provide nutrition for a fertilized egg (see Menopause; Puberty). If the egg is not fertilized, the endometrium is shed during menstruation and is slowly replaced in the course of the next menstrual cycle (see Menstruation).

During pregnancy the uterus expands, allowing the fetus to grow and providing it with protection and nutrition (see Pregnancy). Simultaneously, contraction of the large muscle fibers is prevented. When the fetus is mature, the uterus suddenly changes its role and begins to contract in order to open the cervix and allow both the baby and the placenta to pass through (see Placenta). It then contracts tightly to close off the large blood vessels that have been supplying the placenta. After birth the uterus rapidly returns to its prepregnant state, ready to accept another fertilized egg. Reportedly, this is known to have happened as early as 36 days after a delivery. The uterus seems to have almost no function prior to puberty and after menopause, when it would obviously be unsuitable, both mentally and physically, for a woman to have a baby. All these changes in the functioning of the uterus are caused by hormones released from the pituitary gland, and from the ovaries, and by similar substances called prostaglandins, released by the uterine tissue (see Hormones; Ovaries; Pituitary Gland). How these substances interact is still not fully understood.

Position

In an adult woman, the uterus is a hollow organ approximately the size and shape of a small pear. It lies inside the girdle of pelvic bones. The narrow end of the pear is equivalent to the cervix, which protrudes into the vagina; the remainder forms the body of the uterus. This is connected to two fallopian tubes that carry the monthly egg from the ovaries, and the uterus forms part of a channel between the abdominal cavity and the exterior of the body. Special mechanisms exist to prevent the spread of infection by this route

▶ *Pain, joy, and wonder combine in this unique moment, as a new baby safely completes the journey from the protection of the uterus to the outside world.*

Problems of the uterus

PART OF THE UTERUS AFFECTED	NAME OF CONDITION	POSSIBLE SYMPTOMS	TREATMENT
Entire uterus	Absent	No periods, infertile	None
	Congenital malformation (a double uterus or an abnormal division in the cavity of the uterus)	Often no symptoms (when pregnant, a woman may go into premature labor)	Very rarely it may be necessary to do surgery to make the uterus a normal shape
	Prolapse	No symptoms or the sensation of "a lump coming down into the vagina"	Special pelvic floor exercises, avoidance of constipation, weight loss if necessary. Sometimes surgery.
Endometrium (lining of the cavity of the uterus)	Endometrial polyps	Bleeding from the vagina between periods or after menopause	Dilatation and curettage (D & C)
	Endometrial hyperplasia (overgrowth of the lining of the uterus)	Heavy irregular periods, usually as a woman approaches menopause	Diagnosis by D & C followed by a course of hormone pills
	Endometritis (inflammation of the lining of the uterus)	Lower abdominal pain and heavy periods	Diagnosis by D & C followed by a course of antibiotics
	Endometrial carcinoma	Bleeding from the vagina after menopause or between periods	Hysterectomy and possible radiotherapy or hormones, or both
	Trophoblastic disease (formation of placenta in the uterus with no fetus present)	A feeling of pregnancy and irregular bleeding from the vagina	D & C, avoidance of pregnancy until the condition is cured, drugs if the placental tissue spreads outside the uterus
	Dysfunctional (abnormal) uterine bleeding	Heavy or frequent periods, or both, with no obvious physical abnormality of the uterus	Diagnosis by D & C, hormone treatment followed by hysterectomy if hormones are unsuccessful
Myometrium (muscular wall of the uterus)	Fibroids	Often no symptoms—possibly heavy periods and enlarged uterus	If they cause a problem, fibroids may be surgically removed (myomectomy) or a hysterectomy may be performed
	Sarcoma (cancerous form of fibroid)	Often no symptoms—sometimes the uterus becomes enlarged	Hysterectomy and radiotherapy
	Adenomyosis (endometrial tissue deposited inside the muscular layers of the uterus)	Painful, heavy periods	May be treated by hormonal therapy but often only diagnosed by a hysterectomy
Cervix	Polyp	Often no symptoms—sometimes vaginal bleeding after sexual intercourse or between periods	D & C and removal of polyp
	Erosion or ectropion (cells which normally line the cervix begin to grow on the outside)	Often no symptoms—sometimes a watery discharge	No treatment needed, but the area may be burned so that new cells form (cautery)
	Cervical dysplasia (abnormal cells which may revert to normal or become cancerous)	Abnormal cervical smear	Repeated cervical smears, colposcopy, and occasionally removal of the area of abnormal cells
	Cancer of the cervix	Bleeding from the vagina after sexual intercourse and between periods	Radiotherapy and sometimes hysterectomy

I have a retroverted uterus. Can I still get pregnant?

A retroverted uterus tilts backward from its attachment at the top of the vagina instead of forward (an anteverted uterus). This is quite normal and occurs in about 20 percent of women with no ill effect. There is certainly no evidence that you will be less fertile. Rarely, however, a disease such as endometriosis or pelvic infection will cause a normal anteverted uterus to become retroverted. These diseases can cause a decrease in a woman's fertility, and since they are associated with a retroverted uterus, it is sometimes said that retroversion of the uterus causes infertility. A problem like endometriosis can be treated by surgery or hormone therapy, which does not always cure the retroversion but will improve the woman's chances of conceiving.

Is it true that some women have two uteri?

During the development of the uterus in the fetus, two ducts, called the Müllerian ducts, fuse. This happens about the 65th day of pregnancy, and the fused portion forms the uterus. Occasionally the fusion of the ducts is incomplete, and the woman may have an abnormality such as a dimple at the top of the uterus or two separate uteri, which is rare. Women with this problem seldom have difficulty in becoming pregnant, but they are more likely to have miscarriages or go into premature labor.

Is it possible for a baby girl to have a period?

Estrogen and progesterone can cross the placenta from the mother to stimulate the growth of the lining of the uterus in the developing fetus. Once the baby is born the levels of hormones in the baby's blood rapidly fall, and she sheds the lining, which shows as a pink stain in the diaper a few days after birth. This does not occur again until puberty.

NORMAL CHANGES IN THE UTERUS

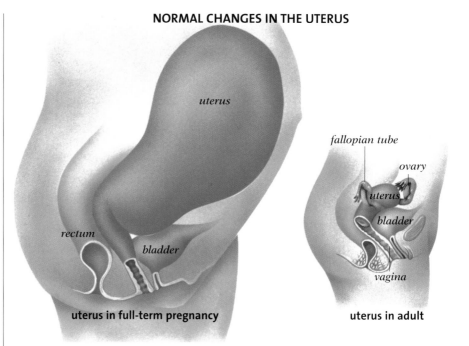

uterus

fallopian tube

ovary

uterus

bladder

rectum

bladder

vagina

uterus in full-term pregnancy

uterus in adult

▲ *The adult nonpregnant uterus is usually tilted forward at an angle of about 90° to the vagina; its muscular walls are thick and its cavity is a mere slit. In pregnancy, the walls expand dramatically to accommodate the fetus and the amniotic sac.*

into the abdominal cavity; the lining of the uterus is shed when a woman menstruates; the cervix secretes antibodies; and the acidity of the vagina inhibits the growth of bacteria.

The anterior (front) of the uterus sits on the bladder and the posterior (back) lies near the rectum. The uterus is normally supported inside the pelvis by the pelvic floor muscles, and by bands of connective tissue and blood vessels from the side wall of the pelvis, which are attached to the cervix (see Pelvis).

During pregnancy the uterus enlarges so that by the 12th week it can just be felt inside the abdominal cavity above the pubic bone. At about 38 weeks it usually reaches the lower end of the rib cage, and about two weeks after the baby is born the uterus can normally no longer be felt in the abdomen. After menopause, the uterus shrinks, but not to its former size. These size variations are controlled by sex hormones, which also control the nature of the glandular tissue lining the uterus (the endometrium).

▼ *It is astonishing that a baby of 8 lb. (3.5 kg) or more could grow inside this organ, which is normally about 3 in. (7.5 cm) long.*

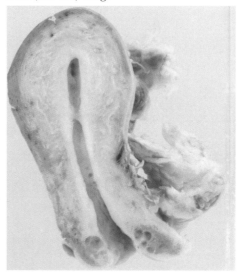

During the first half of the menstrual cycle, the endometrium increases in thickness until an egg is released, then stops growing and begins to secrete substances rich in nutrients to allow growth of the egg should it be fertilized; if it is not fertilized, the endometrium is shed during menstruation.

Congenital variations

During the development of the female reproductive organs in the fetus, two tubes of tissue, called Müllerian ducts, grow from the side wall of the abdominal cavity and meet centrally. These tubes continue to grow downward until they fuse with tissue that will later form the lower vagina. The upper portions of these tubes become the fallopian tubes, and the lower central portions fuse to form the uterus and upper vagina (see Vagina). Very rarely, both Müllerian ducts fail to form, with the result that an adult woman

NORMAL CHANGES IN THE UTERUS

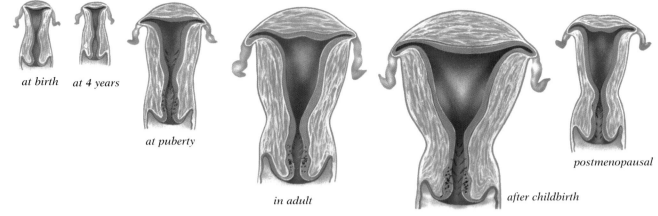

at birth *at 4 years*

at puberty

in adult

after childbirth

postmenopausal

▲ *In a female fetus, the growth of the uterus accelerates during the last two months before birth, probably owing to the high level of maternal hormones present. Within a few days of birth the uterus shrinks, and it remains static until a year or two before the menarche, when the ovaries start to produce hormones. These stimulate the uterus to grow, so that by the time a girl is about 15, it has reached adult size. Pregnancy enlarges the uterus but it shrinks again after menopause. The adult nonpregnant uterus is usually tilted forward at an angle of about 90 degrees to the vagina; its muscular walls are thick and its cavity is a mere slit. In pregnancy, the walls expand to accommodate the fetus and the amniotic sac.*

will have a short vagina and no uterus or fallopian tubes. Nothing can be done to cure this condition, although sometimes surgery is performed to lengthen the vagina. Such women are infertile and do not menstruate (see Infertility).

If only one of the Müllerian ducts develops, the woman will have a uterus and vagina but only one fallopian tube. This does not cause any major problems.

▼ *During the menstrual cycle, the lining of the uterus thickens and becomes rich in nutrients (left). It disintegrates and sloughs off during menstruation (right).*

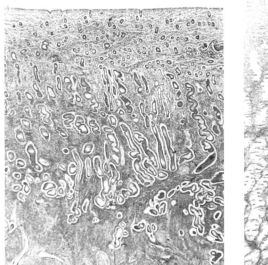

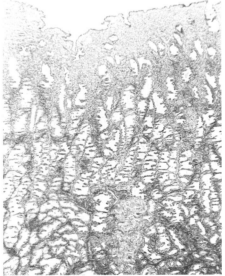

Another rare occurrence during fetal development is incomplete fusion of the Müllerian ducts. This may result in any abnormality from a double uterus to a small dimple at the top of the uterus. If such abnormalities create difficulties for the woman in carrying a pregnancy to term, plastic surgery can be performed to re-form the uterus into a single cavity.

Considering the complex mechanisms that control the normal functioning of the uterus, it is remarkable how few women have any problems. Several different conditions can give rise to the same symptoms as menstruation. For example, bleeding from the vagina between periods or after intercourse is often due to a minor condition such as a polyp, which can be easily treated (see Polyps). However, such symptoms may be caused by uterine cancer, which can be completely cured if it is detected early enough. For this reason, it is very important for any woman who has these symptoms to promptly seek her gynecologist's advice.

Treatment

Abnormalities in the uterine cavity are difficult to diagnose because a direct examination is not possible; a woman may need to have a dilatation and curettage (D & C) to diagnose the cause of a menstrual problem or vaginal bleeding after menopause (see Dilatation and Curettage). Once a correct diagnosis has been made, a doctor can then prescribe appropriate antibiotic drugs or hormones.

Doctors, however, are not always able to control all abnormal menstrual symptoms in this way. Sometimes, the patient and the doctor may agree that the only cure is a hysterectomy. This will stop a woman from having any more periods, and will also make her infertile, but should not otherwise alter her life. However, modern medical therapies are improving and this operation is being performed less frequently. It is hoped that in the future most problems of the uterus will be treated simply with medication.

See also: **Gynecology; Hysterectomy**

Vaccinations

Like many medical advances, vaccination developed almost by accident—when a doctor discovered that inoculation with cowpox virus prevented smallpox. Now vaccines offer complete protection against many diseases.

After he was given a measles shot, my son got a rash and a mild cold. Are these the usual symptoms of measles?

Yes. The measles vaccine, like many of the really successful vaccines, consists of an attenuated (weakened) strain of the virus itself, which is given as an injection of live virus. This is likely to produce the minor reaction that your son had; a mini-attack of the disease. Anyone who has seen the misery of a young child with measles would be the first to agree that the mild reaction to a measles shot is preferable to suffering the disease.

When my daughter was due to get a TB vaccination, the hospital ran a test and said that she didn't need the vaccine at all. Why not?

Tuberculosis is an unusual infection. It is common for people to acquire the illness toward the end of childhood. When this happens, a child may show no symptoms, and build up an immunity that keeps the disease in check. A child in this situation will not need the vaccination, since he or she already has immunity. The original test injection is an extract of the cell wall of the bacteria, and it is read two days later. A red welt on the site of the injection is evidence of a previous tuberculosis infection.

How is a vaccine weakened so that the germs build up immunity and yet do not cause the disease?

Antivirus vaccines are used in a live form, that is, living viruses are injected into the patient, so they must belong to a strain that gives immunity without causing serious disease. The strains are produced by growing repeated cultures of the virus or by infecting and reinfecting a series of animals until the virus has lost virulence.

The development and use of vaccines have revolutionized treatment of many serious diseases. For example, with the help of an effective vaccine one killer disease—smallpox—has been eradicated worldwide, and another potentially fatal disease, diphtheria, has all but disappeared from developed areas of the world (see Diphtheria; Smallpox).

The body's defense system

The body's first line of defense is the skin, which cannot be crossed unless it is broken. The lining membrane of the gut and the lungs are also constantly assaulted by organisms, and their main protection lies in mucus-secreting glands (see Mucus). The final line of defense is the complex, blood-based immune system, which comes into action if the skin or a mucous membrane is breached by a foreign organism.

One of the main functions of the immune system is the activity of antibodies, which are protein molecules that are carried in a dissolved form in the blood (see Blood). The function of antibodies is to help to control and bind infecting organisms, which can then be attacked by phagocytes. Lymphocytes also play a role: they are white blood cells involved in making antibodies and include cells that attack organisms directly, giving rise to cellular immunity (see Immune System).

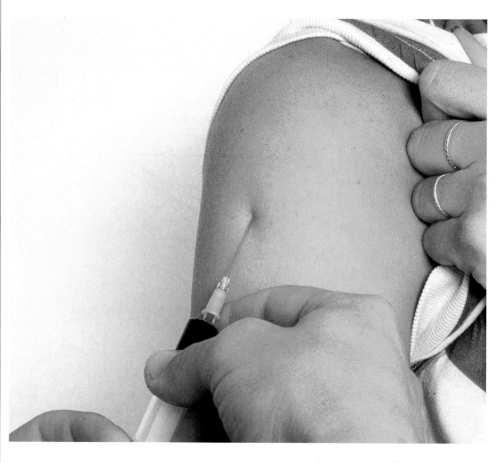

▲ *Vaccination introduces an infectious organism into the body. Although the organism is harmless it stimulates the production of antibodies against the organism.*

Cellular immunity is an important process for dealing with organisms that are capable of infiltrating the cells; one example of such an organism is the tuberculosis bacillus (see Tuberculosis).

Vaccines work by priming the immune system for invasion by an infecting organism so that the body's defenses are prepared for an actual attack by the disease. Generally vaccines are better at building up antibodies than they are at establishing cellular immunity.

The origin of vaccination

Like many of the great advances of medicine, vaccination was an accepted technique before its theoretical basis was understood. In the late 1700s, the English surgeon Edward Jenner heard that milkmaids who suffered from cowpox seemed to have a degree of immunity against smallpox, and he reasoned correctly that this might point to a way of preventing the latter disease. He proceeded to inject the fluid from the pustules of cowpox into

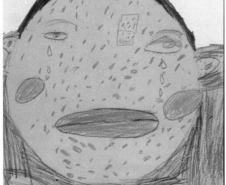

▲ *Variations on the theme of public health: the poster is part of a campaign to persuade parents to have their children inoculated against measles.*

people who were at risk from smallpox. His reasoning was shown to be correct. (Cowpox is called vaccinia, hence "vaccination.")

The reason the cowpox fluid was effective was that the vaccinia virus is so similar to the smallpox virus that it creates effective antibodies to smallpox without giving rise to serious disease. Jenner's intuition occurred long before doctors were aware of antibodies.

Live vaccines

The vaccinia virus is alive, and in certain conditions it may cause serious disease. For example, people with eczema may contract a fatal infection from vaccinia if they have been vaccinated. In most cases, however, vaccinia is a virus that is attenuated for the average individual: that is, it does not normally cause serious disease. In order to

▼ *A medical team vaccinates villagers in Democratic Republic of the Congo in an attempt to control diseases endemic in that part of the world.*

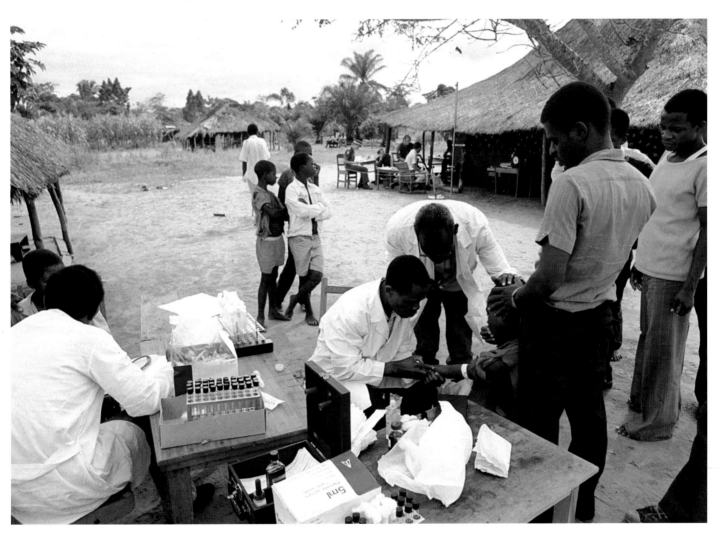

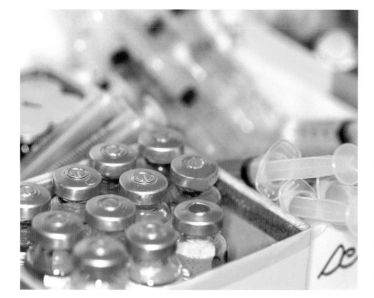

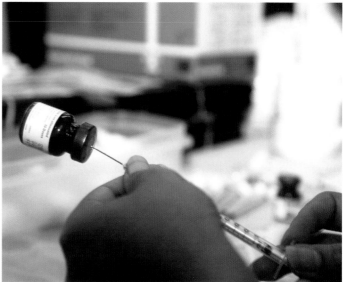

▲ *A supply of vaccine is ready to be used to provide protection against disease. Since the introduction of immunization programs, many diseases have declined.*

▲ *Some diseases may eventually be eradicated if a program of vaccination is implemented. Vaccination is often used to prevent disease from spreading in a community.*

provide adequate protection in other serious diseases such as polio, rubella, yellow fever, and the like, the original virulent (disease-producing) virus has to be treated in the laboratory to reduce its virulence, while its capacity to create immunity is preserved. Virulence is reduced by growing repeated generations of viruses on a suitable medium, or infecting and reinfecting animals such as mice, until the virus loses its capacity to cause serious disease (see Rubella; Yellow Fever).

Killed vaccines versus live vaccines

In some cases, particularly bacterial infections, it is not possible to produce live vaccines—dead bacterial extracts are used instead. Vaccines used against whooping cough and cholera are examples of killed vaccines.

Generally, however, live vaccines are superior to using extracts of killed organisms. In addition, a vaccine such as the polio vaccine can be administered by mouth, so that it goes straight to the normal port of entry of the disease, which is the intestine. As a result, local defenses of antibodies can be built up in the intestinal wall.

Vaccines in common use

In most developed countries, preschool children are offered protection against tetanus, diphtheria, and whooping cough in the form of a combined vaccine called a triple vaccine. Oral polio vaccine is also given at this time. A triple vaccine of measles, mumps, and rubella is given between the ages of 12 months and 15 months; a booster is given between four and six years. It may also be given later.

Travelers may be offered vaccines to prevent yellow fever, typhoid, and cholera (see Infection and Infectious Diseases). Some countries require certificates of immunization against these diseases; travelers should check with a consulate or travel agent.

▼ *A flu shot is given to an elderly patient. The flu vaccination is recommended for those who are likely to become seriously ill if they develop influenza.*

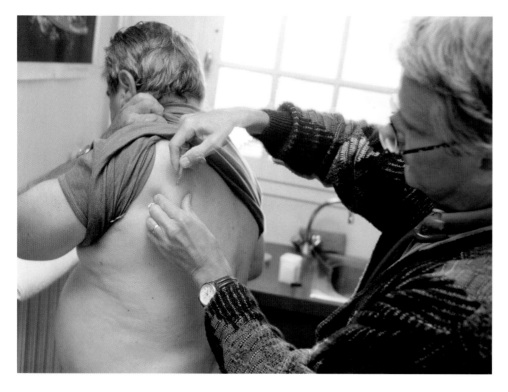

See also: **Immunization**

Vagina

Questions and Answers

Can using a vaginal douche after intercourse prevent pregnancy?

No. Scientists have shown that sperm can swim from the vagina into the uterus (womb) within 90 seconds. This is far too rapid to make a vaginal douche effective.

Is a vaginal discharge normal, or does it show something is wrong?

All women have some vaginal discharge during their fertile years; the amount varies from woman to woman. The discharge also increases at certain times—such as when a woman ovulates or feels sexually aroused, or during pregnancy. However, certain types of discharge do indicate an infection. Women should seek medical advice if the discharge is thin, foamy, and foul-smelling; if it is thick and white; or if it causes soreness or irritation.

During the recent birth of my daughter, my vagina tore and needed stitches. How long should I wait before I have intercourse?

These tears usually take between three and six weeks to heal. You could examine yourself to see if there is any tender area, and if the tear feels healed, then you could attempt sexual intercourse. However, remember to use contraception unless you want another baby soon; some women have become pregnant again as early as 36 days after giving birth.

Could a cyst at the entrance of my vagina be a sign of cancer?

This is very unlikely. It is probable that a duct from the Bartholin's gland has become blocked. Although you should see your gynecologist, the cyst does not necessarily need treatment. However, if it is uncomfortable, it can be cured by minor surgery.

Part of a woman's genitalia, the vagina is the passage for the creation of life, for giving birth, and for sexual pleasure. Although it is prone to some minor disorders, most can be treated easily if medical advice is sought promptly.

The vagina is the channel that leads from the vulva to the uterus. During a woman's life the vagina undergoes several changes. A child's vagina is smaller than that of a mature woman. The lining of the wall of the vagina is also thinner in a child or postmenopausal woman than in a woman in the reproductive years of her life. These changes are influenced largely by a group of hormones called estrogens, which are released by the ovaries.

The vagina plays an important role during intercourse and childbirth. The role during childbirth is relatively passive: the vagina forms the lower portion of the birth canal and is capable of opening sufficiently to allow the birth of the baby. It is only relatively recently that the vaginal changes during sexual intercourse have been described fully.

The vagina is a canal 2¾ inches (7 cm) to 3½ inches (9 cm) long. It is surrounded by fibrous and muscular tissue, and is lined with a layer of cells called squamous epithelium (see Cells and

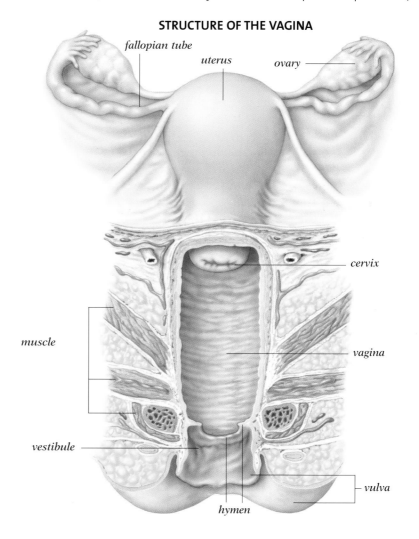

STRUCTURE OF THE VAGINA

fallopian tube

uterus

ovary

cervix

muscle

vagina

vestibule

hymen

vulva

▲ *The vagina is a tough muscular canal situated between the uterus and the vulva. Its corrugated structure is designed specifically to give it the elasticity necessary to allow the passage of the baby during childbirth.*

Questions and Answers

Does a woman's vagina become smaller after menopause, and can this reduce sexual enjoyment?

After menopause the vagina ceases to have a high estrogen level—the hormone that seems to be responsible for its elastic properties and the thickness of the lining wall. This may cause the vagina to become narrower and more rigid, especially if the woman stops having regular sexual intercourse. However, it is seldom a problem if she continues to have regular coitus.

How long after giving birth can you have a diaphragm fitted?

It takes about six weeks after the birth of a baby for the birth canal, including the vagina, to return to its normal prepregnancy state. A diaphragm cannot be fitted until after this time.

Are vaginal deodorants necessary, or can they be harmful?

Simple practices such as regular showers and clean underwear are adequate hygiene measures. Vaginal deodorants can cause a reaction in some women, resulting in a heavier, more unpleasant vaginal discharge than normal. If a woman suffers from an unpleasant, foul-smelling vaginal discharge she should consult her gynecologist rather than use a deodorant.

Can an abnormal vaginal discharge be a symptom of gonorrhea or syphilis in a woman?

Discharge is a common symptom in the early stages of gonorrhea. It should not be ignored, since a reduction in the discharge often means the infection is spreading to other organs to produce pelvic inflammatory disease. Syphilis does not cause a discharge and may go undetected, since the initial symptom is painless ulcers on the genitalia. Most women learn they have syphilis only when their partners are diagnosed.

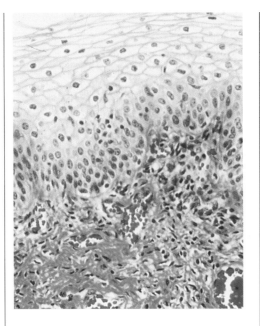

▲ *The vagina is lined with a layer of cells called squamous epithelium. During sexual intercourse, it is lubricated by secretions that seep through these cells.*

Maintaining good health

Take a bath or shower every day
Change your underwear daily
Wear only cotton underwear
Never wear nylon panty hose directly against your skin
Avoid tight pants and jeans
After urinating, always wipe from front to back
Never use douches or vaginal deodorants
See your gynecologist if you notice an unpleasant vaginal discharge

Chromosomes). The walls of the canal are collapsed normally and folded onto one another. These properties make it easy for the vagina to be stretched during intercourse or childbirth. The urethra lies on the front wall of the vagina and the rectum lies on the upper third of the back of the vagina. The anus is separated from the vagina by a fibromuscular tissue called the perineal body. The ducts from two glands called Bartholin's glands enter on either side of the outer end of the vagina; the cervix protrudes into the top of the vagina.

Function of secretions

During a woman's reproductive years the vaginal secretions are slightly acidic, and this acidity tends to inhibit the growth of harmful bacteria in the vagina. However, during the prepubertal and postmenopausal years the vagina becomes mildly alkaline. In these years bacteria can thrive and occasionally make the vagina sore and uncomfortable, a condition called atrophic vaginitis.

The walls of the vagina are well lubricated with secretions from the cervical canal and Bartholin's glands. During intercourse, secretions also seep through the vaginal epithelium into the vaginal canal. A certain amount of discharge from the vagina is normal in all women. The amount increases during ovulation and sexual arousal (see Vaginal Discharge).

During sexual arousal, a woman's genital organs, especially the labia minora and lower vagina, become engorged with blood, and the amount of vaginal secretion increases. During an orgasm the muscles of the pelvis, including those surrounding the vagina, contract involuntarily.

If a woman is particularly tense or anxious during intercourse, the muscles surrounding the vagina will go into spasm. This makes the vagina narrower and makes sexual intercourse painful. This condition is called vaginismus. It can be cured by help from a psychosexual counselor, but it may take many months before the woman can enjoy sex fully.

Disorders

Some women find it embarrassing to consult their gynecologist about problems having to do with the genitalia. However, because most of the problems are relatively minor and respond to simple forms of treatment women should seek medical advice early before complications occur.

One of the most common problems is an irritating vaginal discharge called yeast, which is caused by the *Candida albicans* fungus (see Yeast Infections). This can be treated easily with vaginal pessaries. However, because it is easy to become reinfected, the woman's sexual partner should seek treatment at the same time. She should also be careful that towels and underwear are laundered thoroughly, since the spores of the fungus can lodge in these articles.

Vaginal disorders and treatment

AGE	SYMPTOM	CAUSE	TREATMENT
Infancy and childhood	Vaginal discharge	Foreign body	Hygiene and antibiotics
Puberty	Failure to menstruate and have regular monthly periods	Imperforate hymen (transverse membrane at the entrance to the vagina that prevents menstrual loss, so the blood is trapped in the vagina)	Minor surgery to incise the membrane
	Failure to menstruate in an otherwise normal female due to absent vagina	Failure of vagina to form in the embryo; usually uterus is also absent	Surgery to make artificial vagina. Patient very unlikely to be fertile or menstruate.
Reproductive years	Vaginismus	Psychological cause or physical causes mentioned below	Psychosexual counseling
	Vaginal discharge	Physiologically normal	No treatment
		Foreign body in the vagina such as forgotten tampon or diaphragm	Removal of foreign body
		Vaginal infection with *Candida albicans* or *Trichomonas vaginalis*	Treatment by uterine creams or pills; also treat patient's partner
	Cyst to one or other side of entrance to the vagina	Bartholin's cyst (drainage duct from Bartholin's gland is blocked)	Minor surgery to remove to allow it to drain (marsupialization)
	Abscess (tender red swelling at entrance to vagina)	Bartholin's abscess	Minor surgery to open and drain abscess. Antibiotics are sometimes prescribed at the same time.
	"Lump coming down in the vagina" or incontinence of urine when laughing or talking	Vaginal wall prolapse	Weight loss and pelvic floor exercises. Fit patients, surgical operation; unfit patients, vaginal ring insert.
	Bloodstained loss from vaginal wall	A very rare cause is carcinoma of the vagina	Surgical removal of tumor
Menopause	"Lump coming down in the vagina"	Vaginal wall prolapse or prolapsed uterus	Weight loss and pelvic floor exercises. Surgery or vaginal ring insert.
	Sore vagina, pink-stained vaginal discharge	Atrophic vaginitis (infection due to nonspecific bacteria)	Mildly acidic jelly or estrogen creams inserted into the vagina to inhibit bacteria
	Pain during intercourse due to dry vagina	Lack of estrogen in the woman's circulation	Use of lubricating jelly or estrogen cream in the vagina, or hormone replacement
	Pain during coitus due to narrow vagina	See above	May respond to application of estrogen cream to the vagina

Another common problem is atrophic vaginitis. This condition often affects women in their mid-sixties and it tends to make the vagina sore and uncomfortable. This occurs because women of this age no longer have high enough levels of estrogen in their circulation to stimulate the growth of the vaginal epithelium. The vagina then loses its acidity, so that the growth of harmful bacteria is encouraged. The condition can be treated easily with estrogen creams or by the woman's inserting a slightly acidic jelly into the vagina to inhibit growth of the bacteria.

See also: **Estrogen; Gynecology; Hormones; Intercourse; Menopause; Orgasm; Sexual dysfunction**

Vaginal discharge

Questions and Answers

Is it true that it is normal to have some vaginal discharge?

Yes. A small amount of vaginal discharge is normal. It is merely the secretion of some of the mucus glands in the cervix, together with cells cast off by the lining of the vagina, mixed with a watery fluid.

My discharge is creamy in color. Can this be normal?

If the discharge is slight and nonoffensive and your doctor says it's normal, it is nothing to worry about. It is caused by cells from the lining of the vagina and it is normal for these to be shed. However, if the discharge persists or has an unpleasant odor, tell your doctor.

I find that the discharge varies from time to time. Does this indicate an abnormality?

No, not necessarily. It is normal for there to be a cyclical variation in the normal discharge. It is usually heavier just before a menstrual period, and often the discharge contains an increased amount of mucus from the cervix at the time of ovulation.

My 11-year-old daughter has some vaginal discharge. Is this abnormal?

Prepubescent girls can get a normal vaginal discharge, but you must take her to the doctor immediately. The condition is most likely to be a bout of thrush, which is a yeast organism that thrives in the vagina. Normally, the growth of the organism is suppressed by vaginal bacteria; however, antibiotics can destroy these bacteria and allow thrush to occur. Thrush can be cleared up quickly with antifungal cream and by careful hygiene.

There are many different causes of vaginal discharge, some trivial, some potentially serious, and an awareness of the significance of these can have great importance for health.

Most women are aware that a moderate degree of vaginal discharge is normal, and are not unduly worried by it. The lining of the vagina is almost identical to moist skin (see Vagina), and like skin it is a stratified epithelium and must get rid of surface cells that are cast off. It is these cells that cause the normal whitish discharge. The lining has no glands and is kept moist by a watery fluid or transudate that passes through the vaginal wall from the blood vessels and tissue surrounding it. A normal, or physiological, discharge is of moderate amount and, at worst, causes minor staining of the underwear. It is odorless, and is clear or slightly creamy. It does not involve any itching or redness in the area surrounding the vaginal opening. Such a discharge may vary in amount at different times in the menstrual cycle (see Menstruation). It is also often more marked during pregnancy (see Pregnancy), and may be increased by the use of the contraceptive pill (see Contraception). The condition often mistakenly described as cervical erosion, in which some of the lining of the womb extends down over the cervix, can also cause an increase in the amount of normal discharge (see Cervix and Cervical Smears).

Abnormal vaginal discharge

Abnormal vaginal discharge is very common and causes considerable anxiety to many women. There may be reluctance to talk about it even to a doctor, but this is unwise, since most causes of abnormal discharge can readily be cured and some may require immediate investigation. The most common but not necessarily the most serious causes of discharge are infective conditions causing inflammation of the vagina: vaginitis. There are several common causes of vaginitis, but three specific organisms cause about 90 percent of cases. These are the candida organism that causes thrush, the *Trichomonas* organism that causes trichomonal vaginitis, and a germ called *Gardnerella vaginalis* that causes bacterial vaginosis. All three organisms are commonly transmitted by sexual intercourse (see Sex; Sexually Transmitted Diseases).

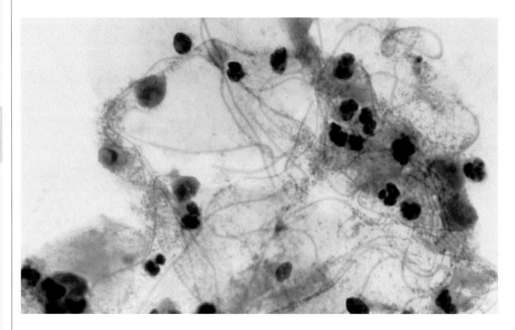

▲ *Using a Pap test, a sample of the vaginal discharge can be used to detect an infection. Here, a micrograph reveals the threadlike Leptothrix bacteria (iron bacteria), which are commonly associated with the protozoan* Trichomonas vaginalis.

Thrush

Several yeast organisms can cause thrush (see Thrush; Yeast Infections), but the most important are the candida and *Monilia* species. Like all yeast organisms, they thrive in an environment with a high sugar content. As a result, untreated or poorly treated diabetes (see Diabetes), in which the urine has a high sugar content, commonly causes genital and vaginal thrush in women. Apart from having the thrush infection treated, all such women must, as a minimum investigation, have their urine tested for sugar.

Thrush, or candidiasis, causes excessive itching around the vaginal area and a vaginal discharge that may be thick and white. The discharge arises because of colonies of the fungus that are partially adhering to the vaginal lining, and that may spread out onto the surrounding skin. A vagina and skin infected in this way will often be inflamed, and the area will be very sensitive.

The appearance is so characteristic that there is seldom much doubt as to the diagnosis. It is not, however, considered good medical practice to rely only on the appearance, and a swab should be taken for laboratory examination and positive identification. Candida organisms can readily be grown in culture, and the microscopic appearance of the typical branching strands of fungus is unmistakable to a microbiologist.

A number of drugs are highly effective in the treatment of candida infections, and these may be applied locally as creams or pessaries. Some of the drugs can be taken by mouth and are given in a single dose.

▼ *Keeping yourself informed about your body can be a lifesaver. If you are generally healthy, a slight vaginal discharge can be quite normal. However, if you suspect you have an abnormal discharge, consult your doctor.*

Trichomonas vaginalis infections

Trichomonas is a single-celled microscopic organism of the type known as a protozoan. It is pear-shaped, and has an undulating membrane along one side and a number of delicate lashing tails at one end by which it moves about actively. A thicker, rapierlike process protrudes from the other end of the organism. Under the microscope the organism is easily identified by its appearance and by its active movements.

Infection with this organism may produce no detectable symptoms or only a minor discharge, but a heavy infection causes a profuse, greenish-yellow, frothy discharge with an offensive odor. It is usually acquired by sexual contact with a male carrier, but can also be acquired from another woman if washcloths or other toilet articles are shared.

The discharge causes irritation in the vaginal area and soreness that may be severe. The organism causes numerous tiny spots of acute inflammation and damage to the lining of the vagina. The result is severe discomfort during sexual intercourse to the extent that the woman may prefer to avoid sexual contact. Vaginitis caused by sexually transmitted *Trichomonas vaginalis* is said to be as common as gonorrhea in sexually active women (see Gonorrhea).

As in all cases of abnormal vaginal discharge, it is essential for a doctor to make an accurate diagnosis so that the correct treatment can be given and the condition cleared up promptly. A discharge is not a sufficient indication of the cause. *Trichomonas* infection is diagnosed by placing a drop of the discharge on a microscope slide, covering it with a thin slip of glass, and examining it under a microscope. In 65 percent of cases of women with trichomonal infection, the organism can also be seen on a Pap test.

Once the cause of the discharge is established, treatment with the drug metronidazole (Flagyl) can be started. This well-tried drug

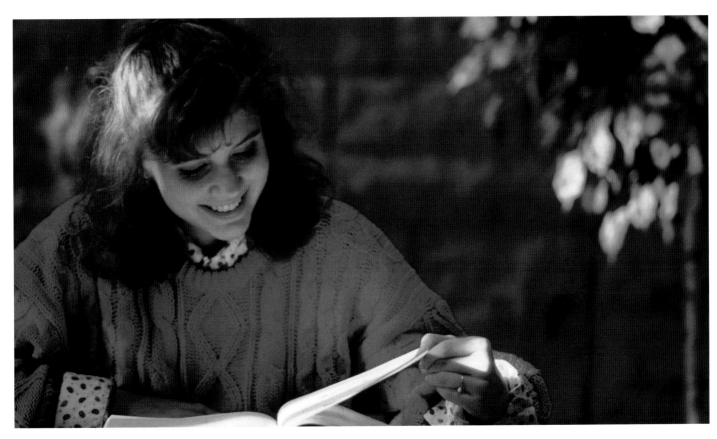

was first approved by the Federal Drug Administration in 1959 for the treatment of *Trichomonas vaginalis* infections. The drug acts by disrupting the helical structure of the DNA of the organism and preventing further DNA synthesis. It is taken orally.

Metronidazole reacts badly with alcohol, and alcohol should be avoided during the course of treatment, which usually lasts for a week; otherwise there is likely to be abdominal distress, nausea, vomiting, hot flashes, and headaches. If a woman has a *Trichomonas* infection, her sexual partner must also be presumed to be infected. If the partner is not given the same course of treatment, reinfection after cure is likely. At least 30 percent of the sexual partners of a woman with trichomonal vaginitis are found to be carrying the organism in their genital tract.

Gardnerella vaginalis infection

The organism *Gardnerella vaginalis*, usually in conjunction with other germs, can cause a condition known as bacterial vaginosis. This is characterized by vaginal and vulval itching and a vaginal discharge. The discharge is thin, is grayish-white, and often contains many small bubbles. Perhaps the most characteristic feature of *Gardnerella* infection is a typical musky or fishy odor, caused by the formation of amines—substances similar to those produced by the decomposition of organic matter. The odor is not claimed to be totally diagnostic of a *Gardnerella* infection, since it is also found in *Trichomonas* infections. It is, however, absent in cases in which the discharge is caused exclusively by thrush. Doctors make use of this effect by adding a drop of 10 percent potassium hydroxide to a drop of the discharge on a microscope slide. The immediate appearance of the amine odor suggests *Gardnerella* or *Trichomonas*. This is called the whiff test.

Trichomonas can readily be seen on microscopy. A more precise indication of *Gardnerella* infection is the presence of what are called clue cells. These are cells from the lining of the vagina that, when viewed microscopically, have a stippled appearance because they are covered with numerous bacteria. Treatment of *Gardnerella* infections is by metronidazole. Again, both partners must be treated.

Many other sexually transmitted infections can cause vaginal discharge; vaginal discharge is a symptom of gonorrhea and chlamydial infection. In both conditions, the discharge tends to be worse in the early stages of the infection. It must be treated, since a reduction in the discharge can mean that the infection is spreading to other organs of the pelvis to develop a persistent condition, pelvic inflammatory disease (see Pelvic Inflammatory Disease).

Discharge from retained material

Occasionally a tampon pushed high in the vagina will be forgotten and retained. The tampon will become infected and will cause a fairly profuse and unpleasantly odorous vaginal discharge. This is one of the easier causes of discharge to deal with, because removal of the offending tampon will soon clear up the problem. Occasionally, foreign bodies other than tampons are inserted in the vagina and forgotten about. Toilet paper has been known to accumulate in the vagina.

Removal of foreign vaginal material is usually easy, whereas a discharge resulting from what are known as retained products of conception (RPC) is not so simply cured. RPC are the tissues of an embryo and its membranes and early placenta that are normally evacuated spontaneously from the womb, an indication of natural

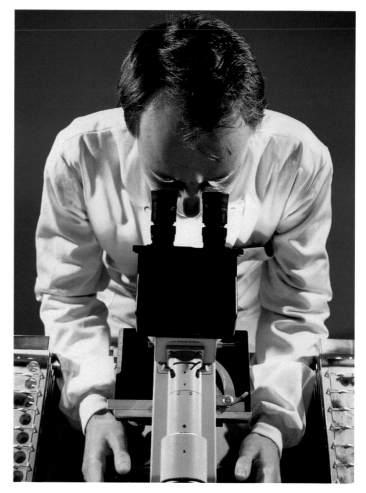

▲ *A laboratory technician examines preparations collected from a vaginal swab in order to detect infections. Abnormal discharges are sometimes malodorous and colored, and occasionally bloodstained.*

abortion of the pregnancy following death of the embryo (see Abortion; Miscarriage). In roughly 10 percent of pregnancies the embryo dies early, usually because of severe malformation. In a small proportion of these cases, the material is retained in the uterus, leading to infection and a vaginal discharge.

The treatment, in the case of an early abortion, calls for a minor surgical procedure known as evacuation of retained products of conception (ERPC). This is done by suction through a tube after gentle widening of the canal of the cervix with smooth dilators. In the case of a missed spontaneous abortion at a later stage, a drug called a prostaglandin, given in a vaginal pessary, and a drug called oxytocin, given in an intravenous drip, will cause the womb to contract and force out the retained material.

Discharge after childbirth

Infection of the raw area inside the womb to which the placenta was attached is luckily rare (see Birth). In earlier times it was one of the principal causes of maternal death following delivery of a baby. Puerperal sepsis killed millions of women before the cause was discovered and proper standards of obstetric hygiene were instituted (see Obstetrics). Since the development of the sulfa drugs, and then antibiotics (see Antibiotics), deaths from this cause have

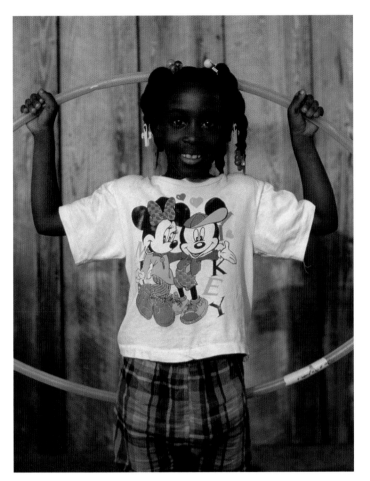

▲ *During infancy and childhood, it is not uncommon for girls to have some vaginal discharge. This is most often due to thrush (candidiasis), which is normally present in the vagina but which is kept in check by bacteria. Antibiotics, poor hygiene, and diabetes can cause the fungus to multiply. Good hygiene and antifungal cream will quickly clear up the condition.*

become very rare in developed countries in the West. Infection of the placental site may still occur, however, and early detection is important. Vaginal discharge is normal after childbirth and is called the lochia. It consists of cellular debris, mucus, and blood. The first indication that anything is going wrong is usually fever (see Fevers), and this may occur within 24 hours of the birth. The temperature may rise suddenly or gradually. Fever after childbirth must always be assumed to be a result of infection until proved otherwise, and must always be reported to a doctor without delay. The diagnosis of puerperal sepsis becomes more likely if the vaginal discharge becomes more profuse, pus-laden, and offensive. The absence of this, however, need not affect the diagnosis. In this context, the vaginal discharge is of minor importance as a sign. Any suggestion of postpartum infection calls for urgent investigation and antibiotic treatment in the hospital. Delay could be disastrous.

Discharge caused by cancer

By far the most important cause of abnormal vaginal discharge is cancer (see Cancer) of the inner lining of the womb (endometrium). This form of cancer (endometrial cancer) is the most common

gynecological cancer. In 2004, approximately 40,320 new cases occurred in the United States. Of these, approximately 7,000 women died, although the mortality rate declined about 25 percent from 1974 to 2004.

Other factors that slightly increase the risk of endometrial cancer include estrogen replacement therapy (see Estrogen; Hormone Replacement Therapy), high blood pressure (see Blood Pressure), obesity (see Obesity), and diabetes (see Diabetes). On the other hand, women who before menopause (see Menopause) used contraceptive pills containing both estrogen and progesterone are at reduced risk of endometrial cancer compared with other women. The difference is very small.

Vaginal bleeding or any bloodstained vaginal discharge after menopause is the most common sign of endometrial cancer at any time during the six to seven months after the periods have stopped. When endometrial cancer is present, a bloodstained discharge occurs in 85 to 95 percent of women. The discharge must never be ignored, and should be reported to a doctor immediately. The fear of cancer is a common reason for avoiding medical attention. The longer treatment is delayed, the more likely it is that the cancer will have spread outside the womb.

In Caucasian women, the cure rate (if the cancer is confined to the uterus) is 95 percent. However, if cancer cells have spread to the lymph nodes in the pelvis the cure rate drops to 70 percent. If cancer has spread more widely to involve the ovaries (see Ovaries) and other pelvic organs the cure rate is only about 29 percent. All three rates are somewhat lower in black women.

It is uncommon for endometrial cancer to spread remotely to the lungs and the bones. Typically, spread occurs by local invasion and by way of the lymph drainage channels. Cancer can spread from the interior of the uterus along the fallopian tubes to reach and involve the ovaries and other pelvic organs.

Cancer of the lining of the uterus occasionally occurs in women before menopause. For this reason, any vaginal bleeding occurring outside the normal menstrual cycle or any new and unusual irregularity in the periods should be reported. Any bloodstained vaginal discharge that does not seem to be menstrual indicates immediate medical attention.

Medical investigation of a bloodstained vaginal discharge involves taking a careful history of the discharge, carrying out a pelvic and general examination, and taking a small sample from the womb lining for pathological examination (see Dilatation and Curettage).

Treating endometrial cancer

The treatment of endometrial cancer is surgery, supplemented by radiotherapy (see Radiotherapy) if the cancer has spread outside the area of the uterus. The results of treatment in early cancer are excellent, and a cure can usually be expected. If there has been wider spread of the cancer, progestational hormone therapy can substantially lengthen life but is unlikely to produce permanent remission of the disease. Eventual recurrence of the malignancy is usually to be expected.

Because of the potential danger of endometrial cancer, it cannot be stressed highly enough how important it is to report a bloodstained vaginal discharge that occurs after menopause.

See also: Pap smear; Uterus

Vagotomy

Questions and Answers

Since I had a vagotomy a few months ago I have had to take medication for severe diarrhea. Will I be on this medication for the rest of my life?

Diarrhea after a truncal vagotomy is a well-recognized complication. It seems to be related to cutting the nerves that supply most of the intestine, and is more common in people who have had their gallbladder removed. In most cases it clears up on its own, but this may take months.

I have heard that some patients who have a vagotomy have surgery on their stomach at the same time. Why is this?

If the vagus nerves are cut at the level of the diaphragm, then as well as decreasing acid secretion by the stomach, the surgery will lead to an inability to empty the stomach. Consequently a drainage operation has to be carried out as well. If highly selective vagotomy is performed, the nerves are cut just as the tiny branches enter the stomach; in this procedure the nerves supplying the stomach-emptying mechanism are spared.

Does a vagotomy affect the heart?

No. The vagus nerve does supply the heart with nerves, and stimulation of these nerves causes the heart to slow down. However, with a vagotomy the vagus nerves are always divided much lower down, after the nerves to the heart have branched off.

I took drugs for stomach acid but now need a vagotomy. Why?

Vagotomy is performed only when acid production in the stomach cannot be controlled by other means; for example, when medication and dietary changes have not helped the condition.

For those people who suffer from duodenal ulcers, a vagotomy often used to be an essential part of managing their condition. Advances in medical treatment have now made the operation less necessary.

The word "vagotomy" means "cutting of the vagus nerve." The vagus are two nerves, one on each side of the body. They are specialized nerves that emerge just below the brain and pass down into the thorax, entering the abdomen through the diaphragm at the side of the esophagus. Each nerve then divides into various branches that supply the stomach, the liver, the gallbladder, and most of the intestines. Branches of the vagus nerve in the neck and chest also feed the heart. The vagus nerves function to regulate the rhythm of the heart and the activity of the stomach and intestines. Stimulation of the vagus increases the output of acid by the stomach lining and relaxes the ring of muscle at the far end of the stomach, allowing food to pass into the duodenum.

Why have a vagotomy?
In the past the procedure was used to treat patients with duodenal or peptic ulcers after, in the early 1950s, it was found that a truncal vagotomy (cutting the vagus nerves at the point where they emerge into the abdomen) led to a decrease in the amount of acid produced by the stomach lining (see Ulcers). However, many patients developed problems with emptying the stomach and a combined vagotomy and drainage procedure had to be devised.

A more recent development, the highly selective vagotomy, is to divide only the tiny branches of the vagus nerve that supply the upper and middle parts of the stomach (the parts that produce the acid).

Developments in antacid drug therapy in recent years, notably the production of proton pump inhibitors, and the recognition of the role of the bacterium *Helicobacter pylori* in promoting stomach and duodenal ulcers, have made it possible to control most peptic ulcers without surgery. Operations are still required to treat serious complications, such as perforated ulcers, but selective vagotomy as a means of controlling excess stomach acid has decreased in the past 20 years.

ROUTE OF THE VAGUS NERVE

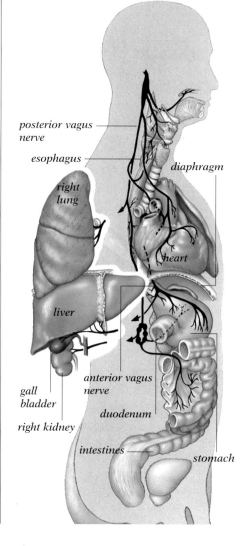

posterior vagus nerve
esophagus
right lung
diaphragm
heart
liver
anterior vagus nerve
gall bladder
duodenum
right kidney
intestines
stomach

◄ *The vagus nerve supplies a number of important organs; the liver and right lung have been lifted out of position to show its route clearly. Performing a vagotomy by cutting or dividing the vagus nerve where it supplies the upper and middle sections of the stomach was once a common operation used to treat duodenal ulcers caused by excess acid production.*

See also: Digestive system; Duodenum; Nervous system; Stomach

Valves

When my father had his aortic valve replaced, he had surgery for his coronary arteries. Is this usual?

It's not uncommon. If there is significant coronary disease both operations can be performed at the same time. Disease of the coronary arteries is very common in the general population, and most people who are investigated for heart valve abnormalities will also have their coronary arteries checked. If abnormalities are discovered, then grafts to bypass the blockages in the coronary arteries are made in addition to putting in a new valve; this results in a better recovery rate.

What is a prolapsing mitral valve and is it a serious condition?

The mitral valve is located between the atrium and the ventricle on the left side of the heart. When this valve prolapses (becomes displaced), blood leaks back into the atrium while the ventricle is pumping. The condition affects 5 percent of women and 0.5 to 1 percent of men. It is not serious and is detected mainly by ultrasound.

I have aortic valve problems but I don't want to have surgery. However, my cardiologist seems anxious that I should. Why is this?

No doctor is going to force surgery on an unwilling person. However, replacement of the aortic valve is a safe procedure in all but the sickest of patients. The reason your cardiologist is so anxious is probably that your aortic valve is obstructed—a disease called aortic stenosis. Not only will the symptoms of the disease be relieved effectively by surgery but, more important, your life may be saved. Without surgery most patients with symptoms from aortic stenosis die within three years.

Although valve problems are no longer the most common kind of heart disease, many people still suffer from them. Because of advances in investigation and surgery, much can be done for patients who are affected.

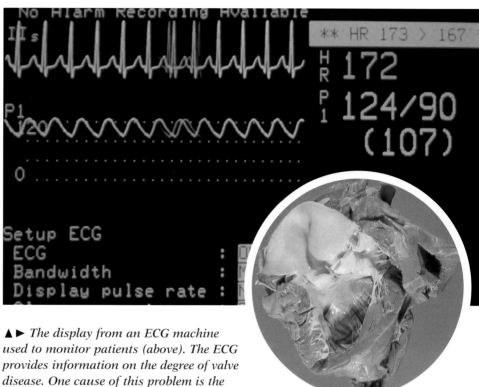

▲ ▶ *The display from an ECG machine used to monitor patients (above). The ECG provides information on the degree of valve disease. One cause of this problem is the buildup of calcium in a malformed valve (inset).*

The heart is a muscular pump and its function is to maintain the circulation of blood around the body. The mechanism is similar to many pumps in that the heart depends on a series of valves to work properly. On the right-hand side are the pulmonary and tricuspid valves; on the left-hand side are the aortic and mitral valves. Changes in blood pressure on either side of the valves cause them to open and close. A closed valve prevents the blood from flowing in the wrong direction.

The pulmonary and aortic valves are similar in structure. They have three leaf-like cusps, or leaflets, and are made of thin fibrous tissue that is nonetheless very tough. The mitral and tricuspid valves are more complicated, though they are similar in structure. The mitral valve has two leaflets, while the tricuspid valve has three.

Each of these valves sits in a ring between the atrium and the ventricle. The bases of the leaflets are attached to the ring, and the free edges touch each other and close the passage between the ventricle and atrium when the valve is closed. These free edges are also attached to a series of fine strings called the chordae tendineae; these strings pass into the ventricle and stop the valve from springing back into the atrium when under pressure.

Problems

Only two things can go wrong with a valve. Either it can become blocked so that blood cannot pass easily through (stenosis), or it can allow blood to leak backward in the direction opposite to the normal circulation (incompetence or regurgitation).

In the past, rheumatic fever was the most common cause of valve disease (see Rheumatic Fever). In cases of this disease, the inflammation affected the valves on the left side (aortic and mitral) almost exclusively, and subsequently could lead to stenosis or incompetence.

VALVES—VIEWED FROM ABOVE

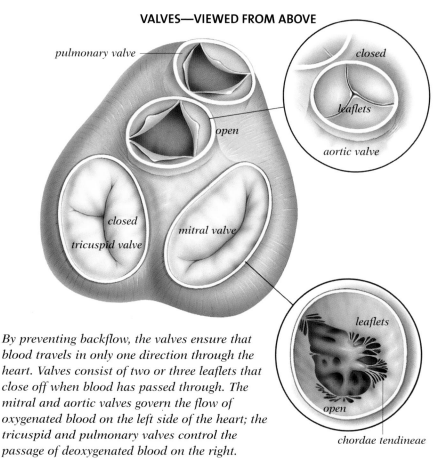

pulmonary valve

closed

leaflets

open

aortic valve

closed

tricuspid valve

mitral valve

leaflets

open

chordae tendineae

By preventing backflow, the valves ensure that blood travels in only one direction through the heart. Valves consist of two or three leaflets that close off when blood has passed through. The mitral and aortic valves govern the flow of oxygenated blood on the left side of the heart; the tricuspid and pulmonary valves control the passage of deoxygenated blood on the right.

POSITION OF VALVES—VIEWED FROM THE FRONT

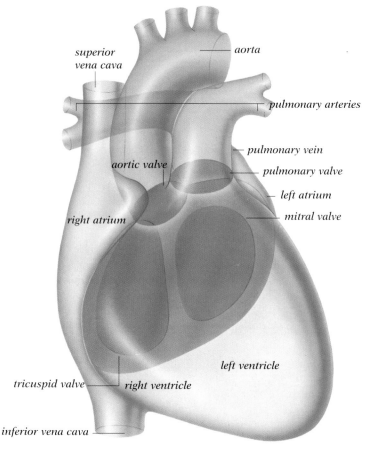

superior vena cava

aorta

pulmonary arteries

pulmonary vein

pulmonary valve

aortic valve

left atrium

mitral valve

right atrium

tricuspid valve

right ventricle

left ventricle

inferior vena cava

Congenital abnormalities are probably the most common forms of modern valve disease. Stenosis or incompetence can occur as a result of minor structural abnormalities of any of the valves; however, the aortic and pulmonary valves are most likely to be affected. Problems may not emerge until late in life when wear and tear starts to put strain on the valve. An abnormal valve may thicken and get deposits of calcium in it over the years, causing reduced efficiency. Abnormal valves also appear to be at risk of picking up germs from the bloodstream, which grow on the valve and start to destroy its substance. This gives rise to a potentially serious disease called infective endocarditis.

There may also be congenital problems that affect many parts of the heart and give rise to problems immediately after birth. One of the most common of these is Fallot's tetralogy: this involves a pulmonary valve obstruction, together with a hole between the two ventricles (ventricular septal defect).

Another abnormality that can cause minor problems is mitral valve prolapse. This happens because there is some slack in the valve and its chordae tendineae, which allows it to balloon back into the atrium, resulting in a leakage of blood.

Symptoms and treatment

Murmurs are usually picked up by a doctor using a stethoscope; aortic and mitral problems may come to light because of breathlessness caused by a buildup of fluid in the lungs. Thickening of the muscular wall of the heart, a result of the extra strain that a blocked or leaky valve puts on it, may lead to heart pain (angina). A final symptom that may lead to diagnosis of valve problems is a disturbance in the heart's rhythm as the orderly contraction of muscle breaks down.

Often the symptoms of valve problems can be controlled by pills, but in some cases surgery may be needed. To decide if this is necessary, a cardiologist will arrange for an electrocardiogram (ECG) and a chest X ray; these give a good idea of the level of strain the heart is under. An echocardiogram, which uses ultrasound to look at the heart, may be performed to picture the valves (see Ultrasound). Finally, a cardiac catheterization procedure may be carried out to measure the pressure in the chambers of the heart.

See also: **Heart; Murmurs of the heart**

Varicose veins

Questions and Answers

Do varicose veins run in families? Both my mother and my father have had them, and I wonder whether I will be affected.

Yes, they do run in families, but no definite inherited link has been identified. All that can be said is that you are more likely to develop varicose veins than you would be if neither of your parents had them. There is not much you can do to stop them from developing, apart from avoiding standing still for long periods.

I have a few varicose veins and I would like to have them treated, but I am planning to have more children. Is it better to wait until I have had all my children before having them treated?

It might be better to wait, unless they are causing a lot of trouble at the moment. Pregnancy does make varicose veins worse, so it would be more sensible to have them treated after having all your children.

My friend has a very bad ulcer on her ankle, and also has varicose veins. Are the two connected?

Possibly. Certain kinds of varicose veins can lead to breakdown of the skin in the lower leg with the formation of an ulcer. However, most people with varicose veins do not have an ulcer, so the two do not invariably go together.

Is it true that some varicose veins can be treated with injections, making surgery unnecessary? And if so, does having injections make it difficult to have surgery later on?

Some varicose veins can be treated by injections. The ones that are suitable are small ones, confined to the area below the knee. Having injections does not affect subsequent surgery, should it prove necessary.

People's upright stance, with all its many advantages, has not come without a price. For many, this price may include varicose veins—those twisted knots of vein that snake embarrassingly, and often painfully, across the lower legs.

Veins are said to be varicose when they become tortuous, irregular, widened, and visible below the skin. The veins in the superficial tissues of the legs are most often affected.

There is no known cause for varicose veins of the legs, but there are many factors that may lead to a worsening of varicose veins if they are already present. Varicose veins run in families, but there is no clear-cut reason for this (see Heredity). They are also much more common in women than they are in men.

The veins
The blood that supplies the tissues of the lower limb normally flows down the arteries to the feet, then back up the veins, and so to the heart. In the lower limb, there are two systems of veins: the deep system and the superficial system. It is the superficial system that is affected because it consists of veins in the tissues between the muscle and the skin, veins that can easily be seen and are called varicose when they become enlarged.

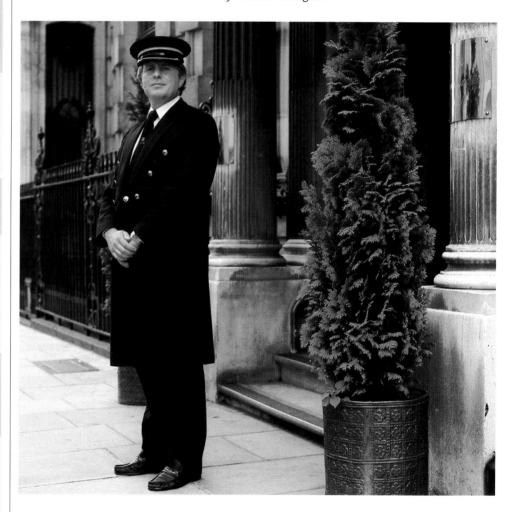

▲ *One might think that a doorman's job is an easy one, straining only his capacity for politeness. In fact, standing immobile for long periods puts him at increased risk of getting varicose veins.*

Can anything be done to treat the patches of tiny purple veins that I have on my legs? They are not painful, but they are unsightly.

These groups of tiny veins, or venular flares, as they are called, can sometimes be helped by laser treatment. A light beam is pulsed onto the veins to seal them and cause them to dissolve. This treatment is usually used to treat only small veins, and multiple treatments are required. Sclerotherapy can also be used; the veins are injected with a medication that causes them to collapse and become reabsorbed.

Is it true that certain jobs can cause varicose veins?

Probably. Standing still for long periods of time increases the amount of blood in the veins of the legs and may worsen varicose veins. However, it is probably a combination of the tendency to develop varicose veins and the prolonged standing that leads to the final outcome. There are many people who have varicose veins who do not stand for long periods, and conversely there are many people whose job entails standing who do not have varicose veins. For those people who do have to spend long periods of time standing, some form of exercise during a break is advisable. Also, while working, make a point of squeezing and relaxing your leg muscles as you stand; this helps pump blood up the veins.

There seems to be uncertainty about whether or not varicose veins cause pain in the legs. Can they? And if so, what sort of pain?

Varicose veins can cause pain in the legs, but usually only if the veins are severely affected. The pain is usually worse at the end of the day, and may be felt at night as a sort of night cramp. It is important that pain in the legs is not automatically attributed to varicose veins, since there may be another abnormality in the leg, such as arthritis or arterial disease, causing the pain.

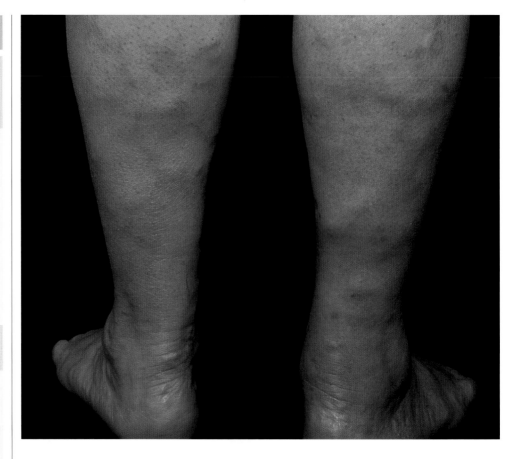

▲ *This photograph shows the unsightly appearance of varicose veins, which are more common in women than men. However, there are many types of treatment available— including surgery, injections, and bandages—so varicose veins can be controlled.*

Both the superficial and the deep veins contain valves every inch (2.5 cm) or so. These valves consist of tiny folds of the lining of the vein, and they allow blood to flow up the limb, but not the other way (see Valves). In patients with varicose veins, these valves are found to be defective. It is not clear whether the defective valves cause the varicose veins, or whether it is the other way around. However, the final effect of having defective valves is that the blood in the vein can flow down the vein, leading to stretching of its wall.

The superficial veins of the lower limb are divided into two main veins, the long saphenous and the short saphenous veins. The long saphenous vein carries blood from the front of the foot up the inner side of the leg and goes deep into the thigh just below the groin. The short saphenous vein carries blood from the outer side of the foot up to the back of the knee, where it also goes deep to join the deep system of veins. The long saphenous vein and its many branches are the most common sites of varicose veins.

Aggravating factors

Although there are no obvious causes of varicose veins there are a number of factors that increase their possibility.

Pregnancy: Many women notice varicose veins after pregnancy. It is probable that the veins were abnormal before pregnancy, but that pregnancy made them worse. There are two theoretical reasons why this should happen. First, the presence of an enlarged uterus leads to considerable pressure on the veins in the pelvis, causing increased pressure in the veins of the leg. This pressure may cause the veins to become swollen. Second, hormones that are produced during pregnancy lead to a general softening up of the supporting tissues to allow the baby's head to pass through the birth canal, and the supporting tissues of the veins may also be similarly affected.

Obesity: Varicose veins can be brought on through obesity because of increased pressure inside the abdomen, together with general weakening of fibrous tissue in the wall of the vein (see Obesity).

REMOVING VARICOSE VEINS

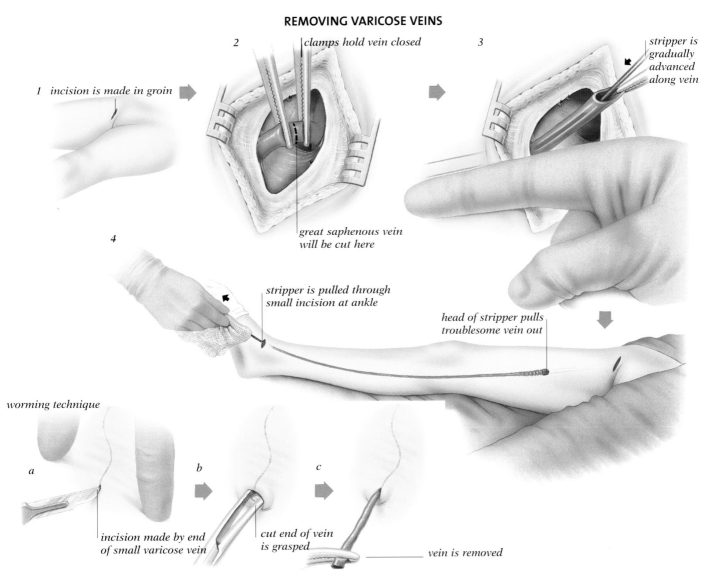

1 incision is made in groin

2

clamps hold vein closed

great saphenous vein will be cut here

3

stripper is gradually advanced along vein

4

stripper is pulled through small incision at ankle

head of stripper pulls troublesome vein out

worming technique

a

incision made by end of small varicose vein

b

cut end of vein is grasped

c

vein is removed

Prolonged standing: Jobs involving prolonged standing may put strain on the veins of the legs, especially if they have to be kept still.

Injury: Sometimes a large varicose vein develops at the site of an injury, such as where a baseball has hit a player's leg. This may be the only varicose vein in an otherwise normal leg (see Bruises).

Deep vein thrombosis: Occasionally, patients who have had a deep vein thrombosis may develop varicose veins in the lower leg, but these are usually of a different pattern compared with the more common varicose veins, which start in the superficial veins.

Effects of varicose veins

Varicose veins do not look pleasant, and by far the most common reason for people to seek medical help is that the veins are unsightly. However, varicose veins can also cause complications and these may necessitate surgical or other treatment.

Because they are thin-walled and near the surface, varicose veins are susceptible to injury. This, along with the fact that the blood flow is much more sluggish in varicose veins, can lead to a thrombosis in the vein. The resulting inflammation around the thrombosis, known as phlebitis, causes pain and redness in the affected area.

Some patients who have varicose veins develop very bad eczema on the lower leg because of stagnant blood (see Eczema). This condition

▲ *(1) The patient lies on a tilt table with the feet raised. The troublesome veins have already been marked on the skin. An incision is made in the groin area and the fascias are divided until the great saphenous vein is revealed. (2) The vein is lifted, clamped, and divided; all the local branches are tied off. (3) The stripper, a thin tube, is then introduced into the groin end; it is advanced down the vein, with the surgeon's finger tracing the vein's path to ensure that the stripper's way is clear. (4) A small transverse incision is made on the inside of the ankle and the stripper is withdrawn through it. Again, the surgeon traces the path of the vein. The leg is raised to reduce bleeding. The worming technique (inset) is used to remove tortuous tributaries. Small incisions are made at sites of uncomfortable veins. Sections are removed using artery forceps. All incisions are stitched, and, finally, bandages are applied to the leg.*

can be treated with skin preparations, but if the varicose veins are removed, then the eczema usually disappears of its own accord.

Treatment

Various forms of treatment have been tried for varicose veins, but modern treatments include surgery, injections, and other remedies, such as the wearing of bandages and support hose.

Surgery: The aim of surgery for varicose veins is twofold. First, an attempt is made to remove the unsightly veins. Second, an operation is done to prevent the veins from coming back again.

The first part of the treatment involves making several tiny cuts in the skin over the veins and removing them a segment at a time. The distance between the cuts will vary, but may be 2 inches (5 cm).

The second part of the operation—treating the root cause of these particular varicose veins—may be more difficult, and it is here that careful examination of the pattern of the individual patient's veins is of vital importance. By examining the patient, first when he or she is lying down and then standing up, the surgeon determines whether the long or the short saphenous vein is at fault, and at which point along the vein the trouble arises.

It is usually found that the valves in the upper part of the long saphenous vein (in the groin) are causing the problem, allowing blood to leak back down the vein. Therefore, if the long saphenous vein is tied off in the groin, the pressure is taken off this vein at points lower down. The blood that would normally flow through the long saphenous vein finds its way back to the heart via a different vein, of which there are dozens in the leg.

This sort of surgery, although it may seem quite elaborate, is relatively minor for the patient. Usually he or she is in the hospital for one or two days and can get up and walk the day after surgery.

Injections: In this form of treatment a special substance is injected into different parts of the vein, causing the lining of the vein to become inflamed. The leg is then tightly bandaged, and remains so

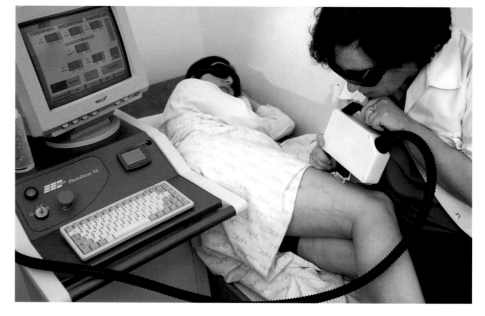

▲ *One type of treatment involves injecting different parts of the vein with a special substance, causing inflammation. The leg will then be bandaged very tightly, so that the varicose vein is compressed.*

for about a month, so that the vein is compressed. The object of the treatment is to get the opposite walls of the vein to stick together permanently, thus effectively closing it.

The main disadvantage of this form of treatment is that it is effective only on small varicose veins, and only if they are situated below the knee (it is virtually impossible to get a bandage to stay on the thigh for more than a few hours).

Bandages: There are no other forms of treatment that are capable of actually removing varicose veins once they are present, but the wearing of support hose can help prevent varicose veins from getting any worse. This hose is specially designed to give firm, even pressure all the way up the leg, and it is usually quite comfortable to wear.

▼ *The modern approach to operating on varicose veins involves making an incision in the groin area and pushing a flexible cable with an acorn-shaped button at its upper end, right down the vein. The top of the vein is cut through and tied to the cable. When the cable is pulled out through an incision at the ankle, the vein is then removed.*

Taking care

If people have varicose veins, the chances are that they will always have a few prominent veins for the rest of their life. Even if a person has the existing veins treated, there is no guarantee that they will not appear elsewhere after treatment. However, there are some things that can be done to try to prevent them from reappearing.

It is important not to do too much standing, if at all possible. Walking is fine, but standing still for long periods is not. When a person is sitting down, the feet should be put up on a stool or chair, so that the blood in the legs can flow more easily back up the body to the heart.

See also: Pregnancy; Thrombosis; Ulcers; Veins

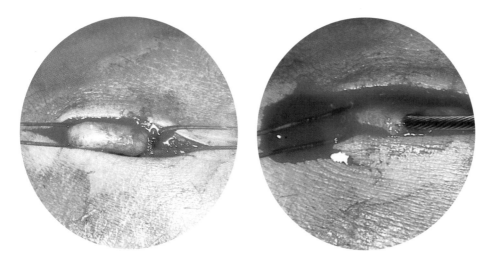

Vasectomy

Questions and Answers

I am thinking of having a vasectomy. Will it affect my virility?

Generally there is no medical reason why a vasectomy should have any effect on virility, or any aspect of your sex life except fertility. A few men experience a temporary slackening of sexual desire after surgery but this is usually caused by psychological factors. For example, it may be due to anxiety about the surgery's having some effect on sexual performance or desire.

How soon after having a vasectomy is it safe to forgo birth control?

Sperm capable of fertilization have been known to survive in the seminal vesicles for three months after vasectomy, but it is usually more like four to six weeks. However, it is important not to rely on these figures; and specimens of semen should be examined under a microscope to ensure there are no sperm remaining in the seminal fluid before you have intercourse without using birth control.

My wife died soon after I had a vasectomy. I am remarrying and my future wife and I want children. Is this impossible, or can the vasectomy be reversed?

Vasectomies can sometimes be successfully reversed, but this is a difficult procedure with no guarantee of success. Surgery involves finding the cut ends of the vas deferens and sewing the various layers together again. Even if this is done there is no guarantee that the internal tube will remain open; and if it is open, sperm antibodies can prevent the development of satisfactory sperm. At present, the pregnancy rate in the partners of men who have had vasectomies reversed is no more than 40 percent.

Male sterilization is one of the most reliable permanent forms of birth control. It requires only minor surgery, but should never be undertaken lightly because there is no guarantee that the effect can ever be reversed.

Vasectomy is a permanent form of sterilization for males, and is an increasingly method of birth control in the United States for men whose families are complete or for those who do not wish to have children. It is equivalent to the operation in a woman in which the fallopian tubes, along which the eggs pass from the ovary to the womb, are either cut, tied, clipped, or sealed off, so that she cannot become pregnant.

Both operations are intended to result in a permanent inability to have children. Because of this, no couple should consider sterilization (see Sterilization) unless they are certain that there is no possibility that they will want children in the future. Before deciding to have a vasectomy it is always advisable for a man to discuss the matter thoroughly with both his partner and his doctor, since there is no guarantee that the procedure can be reversed in the future.

How it works

Sterilization in males consists of removing a section of each vas deferens; this is the duct that sperm (see Sperm) pass along when released from the testes (see Testes). Sperm are manufactured from cells that make up the walls of small tubes (seminiferous tubules) that form each testis. When sperm have matured they collect in larger tubes, the vasa deferentia. These join together and pass out of the testis at the epididymis, a long coiled tube almost wrapped around the outside of the testis. When the epididymis leaves the area of the testis it becomes a long thin channel, called the vas deferens. This is grouped together with the arteries, veins, and lymphatics that supply the testis. Together they form a thick cord called the spermatic cord.

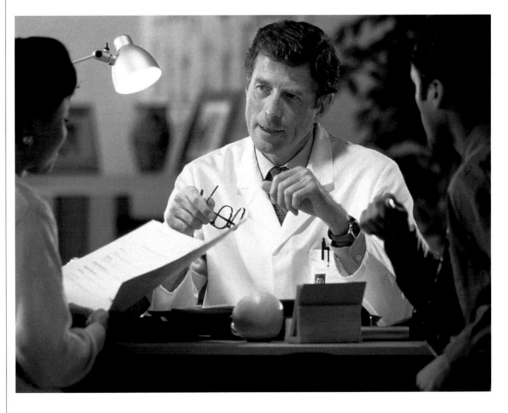

▲ *The decision to have a vasectomy has to be a rational one: it should be made only after a great deal of thought and discussion with both your partner and your doctor.*

Is there a noticeable scar after a vasectomy?

Usually the skin heals so well that you would have to look very carefully to find the scar.

A friend of mine had a vasectomy and he told me that the whole area became swollen and turned blue. Is this usual?

No. Your friend probably developed a scrotal hematoma. This occurs when a severed blood vessel oozes into the scrotum, but this happens only rarely.

What should a man considering a vasectomy bear in mind before going ahead with surgery?

The most important thing for him to understand is that although reversal may sometimes be possible, the operation should be regarded as a permanent measure. He should embark on it knowing that he cannot change his mind at a later date and have it reversed. He and his partner need to be sure that they will not want more children in the future. They also need to be sure that their relationship is stable and likely to last, so that there is no question of the man's wanting to reserve the possibility of having children with another partner in the future. For these reasons, vasectomy is usually the chosen method of contraception for older men.

Have the major Western religions made any pronouncements about their views on vasectomy?

The Protestant church feels that vasectomy is a voluntary matter, but stresses that young and unmarried men should not consider having surgery. The Catholic church is opposed to any form of birth control apart from the rhythm method. The Jewish Orthodox view is as firmly against the procedure as the Catholic one. To date there has been no statement of opinion from the Muslim religious authorities.

From the scrotum, or bag in which the testes lie, the two spermatic cords pass up into the lower part of the abdomen and loop over the lower end of each ureter (the tube carrying urine from the kidney to the bladder) before joining the urethra (the tube that takes urine away from the bladder) where it runs through the prostate gland. At this junction, the newly made sperm are stored in pouchlike structures, called seminal vesicles, until they are required.

During ejaculation (see Orgasm) the sperm, now in a fluid called semen, are pushed forcefully down the urethra and out at the tip of the penis. If this happens during sexual intercourse (see Intercourse; Sex), the sperm are propelled deep into the woman's vagina.

▼ *Vasectomy surgery is simple. Local anesthesia is given; an incision is made in the skin of the scrotum (1). Part of the vas deferens is pulled out (2). It is cut in two places about 1 in. (2.5 cm) apart and the section is removed (3). The ends are folded back (4). The site is closed and the procedure is repeated on the other side (5).*

HOW A VASECTOMY IS PERFORMED

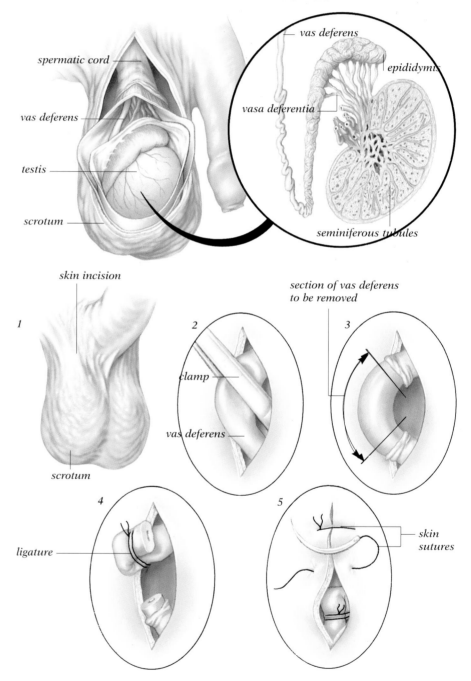

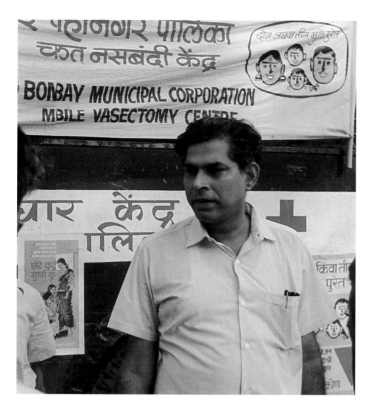

▲ *In India vasectomy has become a controversial issue. Good health education should allay fears.*

There are many forms of birth control (see Contraception). Some, such as the condom and the diaphragm, depend upon creating a physical barrier. Others, such as an intrauterine device (IUD), or coil, prevent a fertilized ovum from establishing itself in the uterus; wherea the Pill interferes with the production of the monthly egg. Sterilization in a male consists of removing a section of the vas deferens, which gives this method the name "vasectomy." The principle is that if a piece of the vas deferens is missing it will be impossible for sperm to pass along it from the testes to be released, bringing about a chance of fertilization.

Advantages and disadvantages

All methods of birth control have their own advantages and disadvantages, and it is very important that individuals choose the one that is best suited to their personal needs and circumstances. Vasectomy, because it is generally irreversible, is a procedure that should be undertaken only after much consideration.

Men who consider having a vasectomy have usually reached their late forties or fifties, they will already have a child or children, feel that their families are complete, and prefer this method of birth control to any other.

Vasectomy has the great advantage of being absolutely reliable and permanent. However, its permanency can be a disadvantage because a reversal of the surgical procedure is difficult and expensive, and, in many cases, impossible.

The decision about whether or not to have a vasectomy should not be made without consultation, although ultimately the responsibility must lie solely with the man. Doctors insist that patients fully understand the procedure and its consequences, and may want to have a signed statement to this effect before they will undertake surgery. Nevertheless, it is also important that a decision to have a vasectomy is taken jointly by both partners. Although the man will have the vasectomy, it will inevitably have some effect on the relationship with his partner. Before planning a vasectomy, a man should discuss the advantages and disadvantages with his partner and family physician.

Surgery

Because the surgery required for a vasectomy is relatively straightforward, it does not require hospitalization, and can be done in the doctor's office or family planning clinic. The vasectomy is carried out under local anesthesia (see Anesthetics).

Two or three small shots are given into the site of the operation to deaden the area. The section of each vas deferens chosen for removal is that part which is most easily accessible and lies at the neck of the scrotum, just below where it joins the rest of the body. A small vertical cut is made through the anesthetized skin and the vas deferens is identified. It is then cut in two places 1 inch (2.5 cm) apart, and the intervening section is then removed. The

▼ *With the aid of a diagram, a consultant at a health clinic describes a scalpel-free vasectomy.*

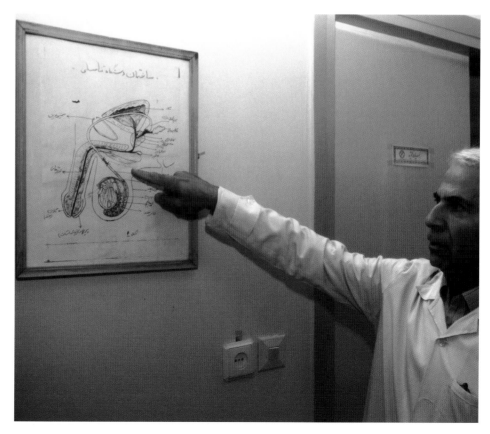

ends are usually folded back on themselves before being securely tied with a material, such as silk, which will not dissolve or disintegrate. The wound is closed with a few stitches and the procedure is repeated on the other side. The whole operation takes only half an hour or less.

After surgery

The wound usually heals in a few days (see Healing), after which the stitches are removed. There may be some soreness when the anesthesia wears off, but this is entirely normal. In a few patients there may be some bleeding into the wound, and this can cause discomfort, pain, swelling, and some discoloration for a few days. Intercourse is likely to be painful for a day or two, and most men avoid having sex until the stitches are removed (see Pain; Swellings).

It is important to realize that there is a substantial time lag between surgery and the time when a patient finally becomes infertile. This is because some sperm are stored at the top of the two vasa deferentia; they have already passed up the vas deferens and escaped before the vasectomy has been performed. These sperm can be capable of fertilization for several months after surgery. Usually by the time three months have elapsed, the sperm should all have been absorbed, but there are cases in which pregnancy has occurred up to three months after a vasectomy.

The exact time cannot be predicted, but it is related to the number of times that the man ejaculates after surgery. If he has frequent sexual intercourse, then he will use up the remaining sperm more quickly. To guard against unwanted pregnancy during this time, other forms of contraception, such as a condom, should be used. It is customary to examine two specimens of semen at eight and 12 weeks after surgery, and if these contain no sperm, then it is considered safe to carry on with unprotected intercourse.

If seminal analysis after six months still indicates the presence of sperm, then the patient should be investigated for the possibility of having two vasa deferentia on one side, one of which has been unnoticed during the vasectomy.

Effects of vasectomy

It is important to realize that the vasectomy procedure is simply an interruption to the flow of sperm into the part where the semen is collected. Even though millions of sperm are released during normal intercourse, they are so small that their total volume will not make any appreciable difference to the volume of semen.

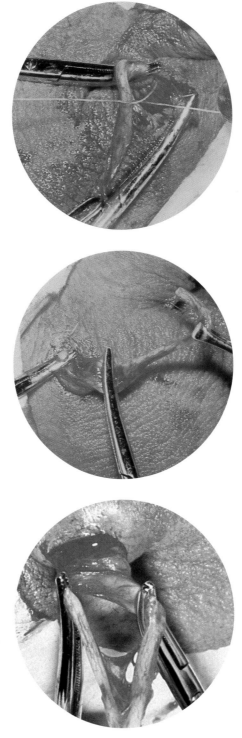

◄ In the later stages of surgery to remove a section of each vas deferens (below), the cut ends are folded back on themselves and ligatures are made. They are securely tied with material that will not dissolve or disintegrate. A reversal of the process, called reanastomosis, aims at the reconstruction of a tube between the epididymis and the seminal vesicle, and is commonly performed on only one side. The ease with which surgery can be done depends on how much of the vas deferens was removed.

The other function of the testes, that of producing male hormones (see Hormones), which are released directly into the bloodstream, is not affected by a vasectomy; nor is a man's sexual drive or ability. A very few men experience psychological problems that do appear to affect their sexual performance, but psychotherapy (see Psychotherapy) or counseling should clear these problems up (see Counseling). In extreme cases, the man may choose to reverse the vasectomy surgically. There is some evidence that tying off the vas deferens on each side can lead to the formation of antibodies against the patient's own sperm. This occurs in very few patients and is of no relevance unless the patient wishes to have a reversal of his vasectomy. However, in this case the main obstacle to a successful reversal is the difficulty of successfully joining up two tiny tubes in the midst of a large amount of scar tissue. The success rate of reversal is around 30–40 percent.

Apart from the occasional case of the development of antibodies to sperm, there are no other known effects. The possibility that vasectomy might cause an increase in the incidence of atheroma (see Arteries and Artery Disease) has not yet been proved by any scientific research or evidence.

Outlook

Vasectomy is almost always completely and permanently successful. In approximately one in 2,000 cases, the two ends of the severed vas deferens do manage to join up again, resulting in an unexpected pregnancy of a man's partner. If this occurs, the man can safely undergo another vasectomy.

Attempts have been made to develop a surgical procedure that would be less permanent, and thus more acceptable to a larger number of men, but no such procedure is available at the present time. Men must be completely sure about their decision before undertaking vasectomy.

> *See also:* **Penis and disorders; Pregnancy; Surgery**

Vegetarianism

Just a few decades ago, vegetarianism was uncommon and considered to be unusual. However, there is now more much awareness of the advantages of eating a diet based on vegetables, fruits, and whole grains.

Questions and Answers

Is a vegetarian diet healthier than one that involves eating meat?

As far as diet goes, eating meat is not harmful in itself. However, eating anything to excess can be dangerous, and a heavily meat-centered diet can, for example, produce too high an intake of fats. However, meat is an excellent source of protein and iron, which the body needs. If these nutrients are not eaten in meat, they must be found elsewhere. The body also needs a certain proportion of fat, so avoiding meat without using careful supplements can be bad for you. However, a well-balanced vegetarian diet can be very healthy, and is prescribed for certain conditions that are caused or aggravated by a high intake of saturated fats or a low intake of fiber. A vegetarian diet is high in fiber and low in saturated fats.

I am newly a vegetarian. What should I eat when not at home?

The best approach is to have the courage of your convictions and tell your host in good time that you are vegetarian. No friend would feel inconvenienced, if you tell him or her early. You wouldn't think twice about stating dietary preferences if you were, say, a diabetic. Your vegetarianism is nothing to be ashamed of.

Will my children get the necessary vitamins on a vegetarian diet?

A vegetarian diet that is properly balanced will contain all the vitamins that you are ever likely to need, if it is carefully planned. However if you are vegan and do not eat meat or animal products of any kind you must give your children vitamin B12, vitamin B2, and vitamin D supplements if you want them to follow the same diet as you. Note that excess B12 is dangerous in children.

Vegetarianism is the adoption of a diet in which plant foods are eaten in preference to, or to the exclusion of, animal products. Knowledge of nutrition increased greatly in the 20th century (see Nutrition). Led by such knowledge and by economic necessity, many Western societies moved away from heavy, meat-centered meals of 10 to 12 courses to a lighter, healthier, more balanced diet (see Diet). The vegetarian movement started in the United States in the early 1970s, fueled by reasoning that growing livestock was uneconomical, and that human dentition was not suited to eating meat. Over the next two decades, other convincing arguments persuaded many people to adopt a vegetarian diet. One of these centered on health issues such as heart disease. In the 1990s the U.S. government introduced a food pyramid, suggesting that the ideal diet should be based on grains, vegetables, beans, and fruits, and that dairy products and saturated animal fats, which are linked to heart disease, should be limited. The pyramid is now more specific and is related to calorie intake, with an emphasis on eating vegetables and whole-grain foods.

Another issue that persuaded many people to become vegetarians was poor animal welfare, such as factory farms, force-fed animals, and calves' being reared in crates to retain their white flesh for those who demanded veal.

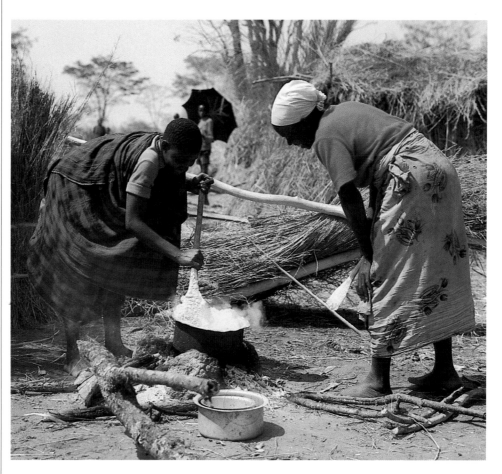

▲ *In the West, vegetarianism is a practice based on personal preference. In the poorer parts of the world, however, the economics of necessity are paramount: vegetables may be all that is available, or affordable.*

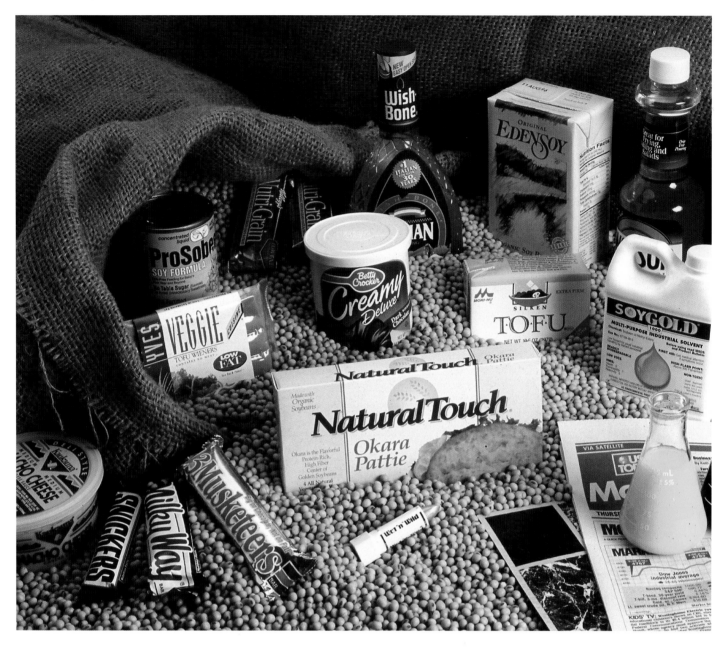

▲ *Soybeans are used to make myriad products; tofu, soy yogurt, soy milk, and soy sauce are just a small selection. Soy protein and soy oil appear in dozens of common foods.*

A way of life

For many people, vegetarianism is a complete way of life that involves more than just dietary rules. Naturism, homeopathy (natural medicine), spiritualism, and yoga all have links with vegetarianism (see Homeopathy; Yoga).

There are many forms of vegetarianism, but most vegetarians fall into one of five main groups. First, demivegetarians at the least rigorous end of the scale are those who will eat white meat, such as chicken or fish, and animal products, such as cheese and eggs, but will avoid red meat. Second are the lacto-ovo (milk-egg) vegetarians, who avoid all forms of flesh, including fish and fowl, but will eat eggs and dairy products. Third are the lacto vegetarians, who avoid all flesh and also eggs, because they believe eggs are embryos and therefore flesh. Fourth, there are those who follow a macrobiotic diet, part of a whole lifestyle based on hatha yoga, which concentrates on whole grains, cereals, and some vegetables, but also includes fish (see Macrobiotics). Last, there are the vegans, who eat no flesh or animal products of any kind.

Why become a vegetarian?

There are probably almost as many reasons for becoming a vegetarian as there are vegetarians. The motive may be ethical, economic, ecological, social, emotional, spiritual, or medical. One obvious and widespread reason is a simple dislike of meat—its taste or appearance, or both. Other reasons are aesthetic: for example, one person became a vegetarian after seeing a particularly bloody automobile crash; she claimed that the mutilated bodies reminded her of a butcher's shop, and that she has been unable to eat meat ever since.

In early cultures, there were often cultural reasons for a vegetarian diet. Some Indian and African communities have no tradition of hunting, and therefore they have no source of fresh

ECONOMICS OF VEGETARIANISM

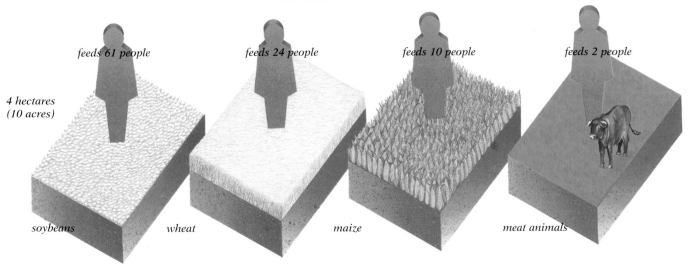

feeds 61 people

feeds 24 people

feeds 10 people

feeds 2 people

4 hectares
(10 acres)

soybeans

wheat

maize

meat animals

meat. Rather, they live on cereals and plants. Economic pressures may also be relevant, since with the rising cost of fish and meat, many people cannot afford to buy either.

Perhaps more commonly, there are ethical reasons for becoming a vegetarian. The Vegan Society was founded by vegetarians who felt that the methods used in dairy farming, especially the early separation of cow and calf, were in some ways more cruel than those of meat production. In protest, they refused to eat animal products of any kind.

Most vegetarians avoid meat and meat products because they are distressed by the idea of animals being slaughtered to provide their food, by the methods of slaughter, or by the treatment of the animals on the journey to a slaughterhouse.

There is also an ecological and economic argument that the starving people of the world could be better provided for if our diet were not so meat-centered. Fifty percent of the world cereal crop is fed to animals, and it takes 10 tons of vegetable protein fed to an animal to produce one ton of animal protein (see Protein). The theory is that if less grain were used to raise fewer animals for slaughter, more grain would be available for humans.

Several religious and spiritual sects advocate vegetarianism as part of a pure, simple life. The macrobiotic lifestyle, for example, centers on the belief that pain and disease are the result of spiritual imbalance, and that concern for the origin of food is one way to restore the balance. A pure natural diet is thought to rid the body of harmful toxins. If a natural diet is eaten and, at the same time, yoga and prayer are practiced, spiritual well-being will be promoted.

Finally, some people become vegetarians for health reasons. Although a meat-free diet is not necessarily better for everyone, certain medical conditions—especially heart and digestive diseases—can be improved by eating a vegetarian diet which is low in saturated fat and high in fiber.

A balanced vegetarian diet

In the 1970s, it was believed that the quality of protein obtained from individual plant sources was low compared with animal protein, and that by combining certain plant proteins a high-quality protein can be obtained. This theory has been disproved and it is

▲ *These diagrams represent how, in terms of land use, it is more economical to grow crops rather than graze animals destined for slaughter and the dinner table.*

▼ *Soybeans are used in many everyday products; for example, soy oil is the most widely used oil in the United States.*

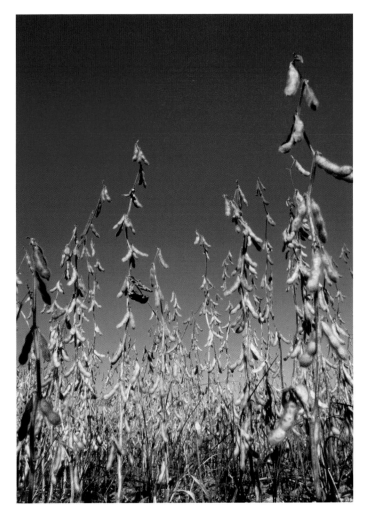

now known that all the essential and nonessential amino acids are to be found in single unrefined starches such as rice, wheat, potatoes, and corn. If people eat enough calories, they are virtually certain of getting enough protein. After all, people were eating farm animals that ate nothing but plants yet remained healthy.

The original myth about complementary proteins seems to have originated from a study on rats. Rats, however, require 10 times as much protein as humans, because rat milk is 50 percent protein compared with 5 percent protein in human breast milk.

Vegans do not eat any dairy products or eggs; therefore, to ensure that their protein requirements are met, they should eat a diet of mixed protein sources, including cereals, nuts, legumes, potatoes, and oil seeds. A balanced vegetarian diet can have many health advantages. Vegans tend to weigh less than omnivores (those who eat many kinds of food—flesh and vegetable), and weighing less can be an advantage. Also, vegetarians eat a greater amount of fiber, which helps prevent constipation (see Constipation) and intestinal diseases such as cancer and colitis.

Other conditions that a vegetarian diet has improved or even cured in some cases include infantile eczema, childhood asthma, acne, and, in adults, diabetes, hypertension, circulatory problems, blood clots, angina, and migraine. The most widely discussed argument for vegetarianism on health grounds, however, is the

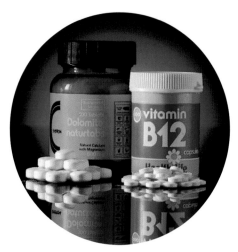

▲ *The crux of adopting a vegetarian diet is that it must be balanced, containing the vitamins your children are likely to need; vitamin supplements can provide reassurance.*

avoidance or alleviation of heart disease (see Heart Attack; Heart Disease). One of the most common causes of heart attacks is the accumulation of fatty deposits along the walls of the coronary arteries, a condition called atheroma. Diets rich in fats—particularly saturated fats (fats with a high concentration of hydrogen atoms), which are found predominantly in animal products—appear to contribute to the disease (see Fats).

Heart disease is almost unknown in nonindustrial vegetarian communities. The highest incidence of heart disease is in Russia, followed by countries in central Europe and eastern Europe. The United States is placed at about number 13 in a world table, near to the UK, New Zealand, and the Scandinavian countries. France and Japan are at the bottom of the table, with a much lower incidence of heart disease.

▼ *These soybean seeds show a wide range of colors, sizes, and shapes. Soybeans are grown in half of the United States, yet were virtually unheard of 100 years ago.*

▼ *A tempting lunch box for kids to take to school. What's special about this one is that the food in it is vegetarian and contains all the nutrients necessary for a well-balanced meal.*

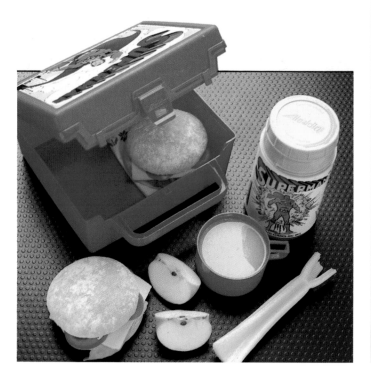

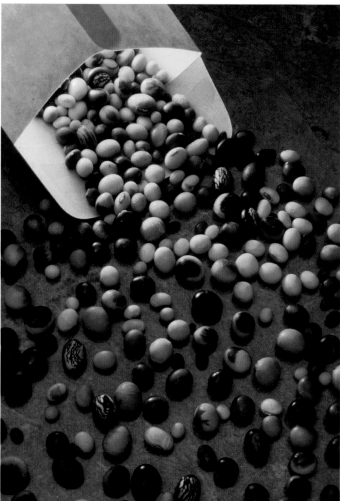

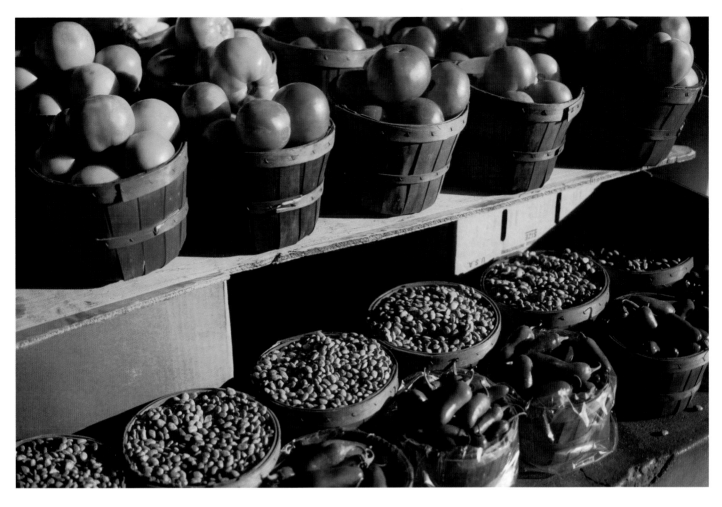

▲ *Fresh fruits and vegetables, and nuts and legumes are perfect ingredients for a vegetarian diet; they can be obtained at farmers' markets.*

A balanced vegetarian diet

A commitment to vegetarianism, and especially veganism, requires a sensible approach to diet, and factors that contribute to good health must not be neglected.

Weight loss, often accompanied by a loss of energy, is a common effect of changing over to a vegetarian diet. This can be serious in someone who is already underweight. More serious illnesses that are connected with veganism in particular are spinal ataxia, a condition causing an unsteady gait, stooped posture, and loss of balance and sensation in the legs; and megaloblastic anemia, a deficiency in the blood (see Anemia). Both of these conditions, caused by vitamin B12 deficiency, are quite rare (see Vitamin B), but deficiency of this vitamin is the major health risk for vegans.

Cobalt is a vital constituent of this vitamin; in a vegan diet, because vitamin B12 is found only in animal foods or microorganisms, it can be obtained naturally only by eating vegetables old enough to have a growth of mold on them. One way to avoid such a deficiency is to include a vitamin B12 supplement in the diet. There is vitamin B12 in eggs and cheese, so it is only vegans who are at risk of a deficiency.

Vitamin D is also absent from plant foods. However, individuals can make this vitamin by the action of sunlight on the skin. Vitamin D deficiency can occur in children reared on a vegan diet if they are not sufficiently exposed to sunlight. It would be a sensible precaution, especially in winter, to give children extra vitamin D in the form of drops (see Vitamin D).

Ultimately, the choice of diet is a personal one, based on belief, preference, or circumstances. However, a properly balanced diet

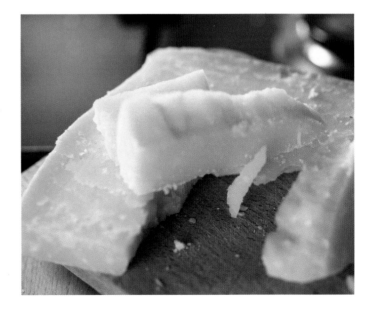

▲ *A small quantity of cheese added to a vegetarian dish enriches it with protein.*

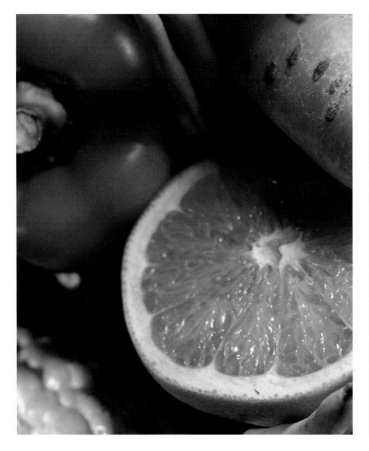

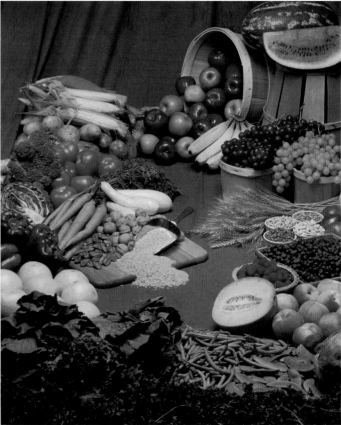

▲ *Citrus fruits are a good source of vitamin C and bioflavonoids, which have a beneficial effect on the body. They protect the nervous system and strengthen capillary walls.*

▲ *The U.S. government food guide pyramid recommends three to five servings of vegetables and two to four servings of fruit daily as part of a healthy diet.*

should consist of the correct proportions of fats, carbohydrates, proteins, vitamins, and minerals, and contain appropriate calories.

▼ *A diet rich in soy and whey protein, found in products such as soy milk and low-fat yogurt, has been shown to reduce the incidence of breast cancer in rats.*

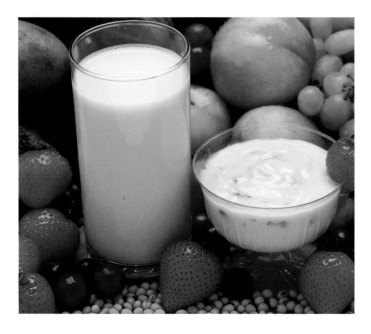

Changing one's diet should always be a slow and careful process, as any sudden change can be a shock to the system. A dietitian should be consulted before making any radical change in the amount or type of food eaten. A well-balanced diet and plenty of sensibly planned exercise are vital for health. Whether that diet is vegetarian depends on individual needs and preferences.

Daily vegetarian fare
A good daily intake of fresh vegetables and fruit is essential, particularly green leafy vegetables. Because cooking can destroy vitamins, minerals, and other nutrients, vegetables can be eaten raw or lightly steamed, baked, or microwaved.

Brown rice, oats, barley, corn, nuts and legumes, and seeds supply adequate amounts of dietary fiber. Because a range of health problems are associated with the consumption of saturated fats, butter and cheese should be eaten rarely. Monounsaturated oils such as canola oil or olive oil can be substituted. Soy products such as tofu supply protein and have the advantage that they do not contain cholesterol or saturated fat. Fats are made up of fatty acids; most are made by the body but two of the unsaturated fatty acids have to be supplied in the diet. A good source for vegetarians is flaxseed oil, which contains omega-3 fatty acids, and safflower oil and soybean oil are important sources of omega-6 fatty acids.

See also: Alternative medicine; Digestive system; Weight

Veins

My father had open-heart surgery recently for his angina, and a vein was removed from his leg. How was this vein used in the surgery?

The vein from the leg is used to form a bypass for the blocked coronary arteries that cause angina. Veins are designed to carry blood at much lower pressure than arteries, but they can cope very well with the extra strain usually imposed on the arteries.

Is it true that you may get clots in the legs if you go on an airplane, and is this very dangerous?

Yes, it is possible. If you are sitting still for a long time, then the rate of blood flow in the deep veins of the legs slows down. This is largely because the muscles in your legs, which are active when you are moving about, also help pump the blood back toward the heart; this pumping is lost when you sit down. There is also pressure from the seat on your thighs as you sit, which will tend to reduce the rate of blood flow. Once the rate of flow falls, the blood clots more easily. The danger of blood clots in the deep veins of the legs is that they can break off and pass through the heart to get stuck in the lungs. You should keep your feet moving when you are on a long flight, and make sure that you get out of your seat every hour or so if possible.

How long can a needle be left in the arm of a patient who is being drip-fed?

Modern needles are nearly all thin plastic tubes called cannulas. A simple cannula in the arm usually lasts only a few days. In intensive care units, where drips may be required for long periods, longer fine tubes called catheters are used, and these can be put into the big veins in the chest. These central lines are designed to last longer than the small cannulas in the arm.

After giving up oxygen and nourishment to the tissues, blood is carried back to the heart by the veins. These specially designed channels play as important a part as the arteries in the efficient working of the circulation.

Veins are similar to arteries in their distribution; the arteries and veins associated with a particular organ or tissue often run together, but there are major differences. Many veins have valves, which the arteries do not, and the walls of an artery are always thicker than those of a vein of the same size, whereas the central channel, or lumen, will be much bigger in the vein than the artery.

Structure and function

Veins are tubes of muscular and fibrous tissue. Their walls have an outer layer, the tunica adventitia; a middle layer of muscle fiber, the tunica intermedia; and an inner lining, the tunica intima. They contain only a thin layer of muscle. After passing through the capillaries from the arteries, blood enters the venous system. It first passes into very small vessels called venules, which are the venous equivalent of arterioles. It then makes its way into small veins and back toward the heart along the veins that are large enough to be seen under the skin. Veins of this size contain valves that prevent blood from flowing back toward the tissues. The valves have little half-moon-shaped cups that project into the lumen of the vein, and these make the blood flow in only one direction (see Valves).

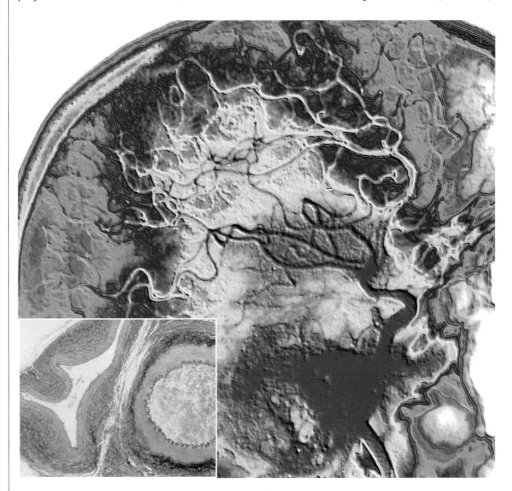

▲ *The carotid angiogram (above)—a type of X ray of blood vessels—graphically illustrates the network of veins carrying blood away from the head. The micrograph (inset) shows transverse sections of a vein and an artery; the vein is on the left.*

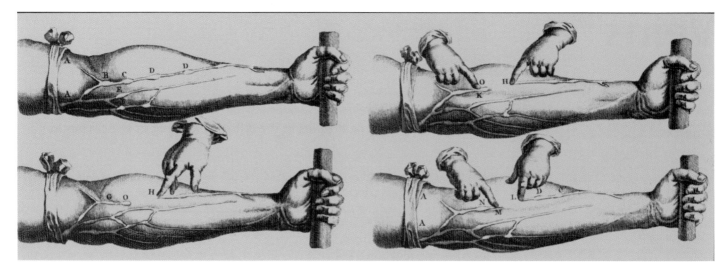

▲ *The English physician William Harvey, who proved that the blood circulates (1628), illustrated how blood in the arm flows continuously in one direction, controlled by valves in the veins.*

Eventually, blood flowing back to the heart enters one of two large veins; the inferior vena cava receives blood from the lower half of the body, and the superior vena cava receives blood from the head and arms. These vessels are about 1 inch (2–3 cm) wide, and they enter the right atrium of the heart. Blood passes from here into the right ventricle, and then into the lungs via the pulmonary arteries. It leaves the lungs by means of the pulmonary veins, which enter the left atrium of the heart (see Lung and Lung Diseases).

Special types of vein

There is one area where the veins are arranged in a very different way from the arteries, and this is in the intestines. Here, instead of draining into a vein that passes straight into the heart, blood from the intestines is drained into what is called the hepatic portal system of veins. This allows the blood, which may be rich in digested food, to be carried directly to the liver.

Once blood from the intestines reaches the liver, it passes in among the liver cells, in special capillaries that are called sinusoids, and then enters the system of veins called the hepatic veins. These eventually lead on to the inferior vena cava, and thus into the heart. This system ensures that food passed into the venous system from the intestines is brought to the liver for chemical processing in the most efficient way (see Liver and Liver Diseases).

Other areas where there are special kinds of venous structure are in the extremities—the hands, feet, ears, and nose. Here it is possible to find direct communications between the small arteries and veins,

VEIN NETWORKS

jugular
subclavian
superior vena cava
coronary
hepatic portal
iliac
great saphenous

pulmonary
basilic
hepatic
inferior vena cava
femoral
popliteal
tibial

◄ *The body's complex system of veins returns blood in the direction of the heart (as opposed to arteries, which carry it away) through the conduits called the venae cavae.*

where blood may flow through from one to the other without having to go through a system of capillaries in the tissues. The main function of these arteriovenous connections is related to the control of body temperature. When they are open, heat loss increases and the body cools down (see Temperature).

There are similar connections between the arteries and veins in the genital areas. These allow for the engorgement of blood that occurs in the genitals as a result of sexual excitement (see Genitals).

What can go wrong?

One serious problem that affects veins is the tendency of blood clots to form in them. This is likely to happen because of the slowness with which blood flows along the veins, in contrast with the rapid flow maintained in the arteries. Smoking and the Pill increase the risk of clotting, although the low dose of estrogen in modern contraceptive pills has much reduced this danger (see Oral Contraceptives; Smoking).

Another major trouble is caused by the upright stance of human beings—this leads to pressure in the veins of the legs, since they are supporting a high column of blood. This can result in twisted, engorged veins in the legs called varicose veins. However, problems affecting the veins are minor compared with those arising from arterial disease (see Arteries and Artery Disease).

See also: **Blood; Capillaries; Circulatory system; Heart; Open-heart surgery; Thrombosis; Varicose veins**

Ventricular fibrillation

Thousands of people who are walking around today have been treated for attacks of ventricular fibrillation. All would have died but for the treatment they were given—treatment that first became available in the 1960s.

Ventricular fibrillation (VF) is a disturbance of the orderly electrical activity of the heart. The fibers that make the heart's pumping chambers start to relax and contract in a totally uncoordinated way, so that the heart is unable to pump blood. Within seconds of an attack, a person will become unconscious and death will follow in a minute or two. Urgent treatment is needed, whether it be from a paramedic team that can get to the patient quickly, or in a coronary care unit.

Causes of VF

The main cause of VF is a heart attack, which is responsible for many of the deaths from the condition. A heart attack usually arises from coronary artery disease, in which the heart's own blood supply becomes obstructed. Other heart problems can also cause VF, particularly those in which there is an electrical disturbance of the heart. This disturbance may eventually lead to various disorders in which the heart beats too fast. In some cases the heart rate is so fast that the heart can cope for only short periods of time before VF becomes a serious possibility. Sometimes the heart is affected by a disease that involves its own muscles—called cardiomyopathy—and in a few cases this may lead to a rise in the heart rate, and so bring on VF.

Mechanism of VF

The regular and automatic beating of the heart results from a very sophisticated timing system that conducts electrical impulses to the various parts of the heart. These impulses lead the heart muscle to contract, and they are ordered so that the ventricles contract after the atria and both sets of chambers have adequate time to relax and recover for the next heartbeat.

In the various diseases that raise the rate of heartbeat, the mechanism becomes disrupted, causing the chambers to beat at a very fast and inefficient rate. In VF, the whole system breaks

Questions and Answers

Is an attack of ventricular fibrillation always fatal?

An attack is likely to be fatal unless treatment is given immediately. This consists of administering an electric shock to the heart to revert its activity to normal. Alternatively, if you thump hard on the victim's breastbone within half a minute after he or she loses consciousness, you may convert the heart rhythm back to normal without the aid of electricity, but the chances of success diminish as the ventricular fibrillation becomes established. A few patients survive without being given treatment because the electrical activity of their heart reverts on its own. As a general rule, however, ventricular fibrillation is fatal without treatment.

My doctor said that I have atrial fibrillation. Does this mean that I am at risk of ventricular fibrillation?

No. In atrial fibrillation the atria of the heart are beating in an uncoordinated way. This has little impact on the overall function of the heart, since the two ventricles are still able to pump. In ventricular fibrillation no blood is pumped through the heart, and death will follow unless the heart's electrical activity is restored to normal. Atrial fibrillation—a common and relatively minor heart problem—does not lead to ventricular fibrillation, so you shouldn't worry.

Is it true that heart surgeons may deliberately put the heart into ventricular fibrillation?

Yes. They do this so that the heart moves less, making it easier to operate on. In heart surgery, where the work of the heart is taken over and carefully controlled using a bypass machine, there is little risk involved. The process can be easily reversed by using a defibrillator, which restarts the heart.

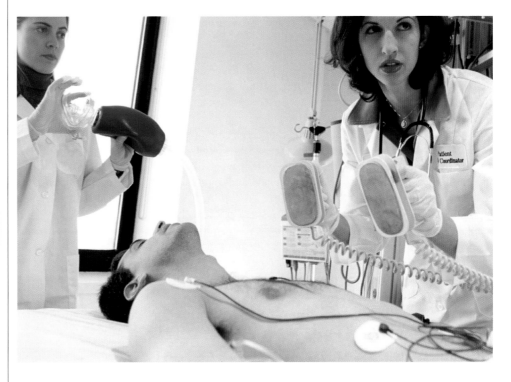

▲ *A doctor is about to use a defibrillator on a patient in an intensive care unit.*

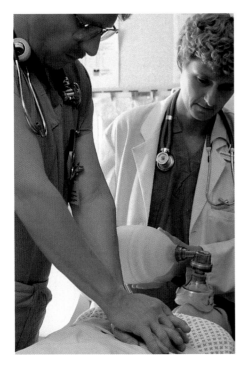

▲ *When defibrillation is unsuccessful in restoring normal heart rhythm after a heart attack, chest compression and artificial respiration are necessary.*

down so that individual muscle fibers contract and relax independently of each other, with no overall contraction of the heart, and no pumping of blood.

THE HEART'S NORMAL PUMPING ACTION

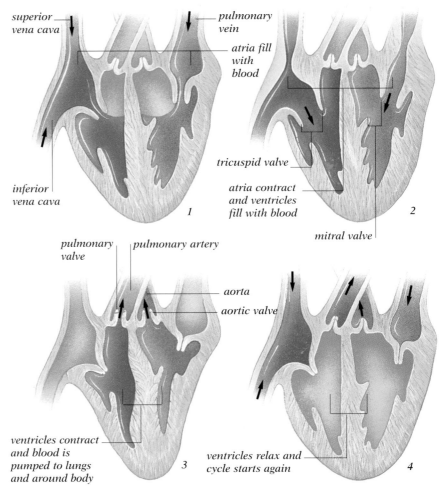

superior vena cava

pulmonary vein

atria fill with blood

inferior vena cava

1

tricuspid valve

atria contract and ventricles fill with blood

mitral valve

2

pulmonary valve

pulmonary artery

aorta

aortic valve

ventricles contract and blood is pumped to lungs and around body

3

ventricles relax and cycle starts again

4

▲ *A number of electrical impulses ensure the efficient working of the heart. They govern the rhythmic and coordinated action of the atria, ventricles, and valves.*

Treatment

The revolution in treatment of VF has been the introduction of defibrillators. They work by delivering a shock across the heart when two electrical pads are placed on the chest: one on the breastbone (sternum) and one at the apex of the heart, just below the left nipple. During heart surgery, two smaller pads are placed on the surface of the exposed heart, and a much lower current is used (see Electrocardiogram).

The basic principle of defibrillation is that an electric shock will cause the simultaneous electrical discharge of all the cells in the heart. This gives the normal conducting system what might be described as a clean slate on which to work, and enables it to reinstate normal, orderly electrical activity.

Defibrillation is not without its dangers. A shock can actually put a heart into VF, although this is a risk only when this form of treatment is being used for less serious disturbances of the heart rate; once the patient is in VF, there is obviously nothing to lose. Further, when defibrillation is performed, neither the patient nor his or her bed must be touched. The electrical pads, or paddles, have insulated handles to protect the operator.

Prevention

Great efforts are made to identify patients who are at risk of VF; one of the main indications is that they have already suffered an attack. Such patients will usually be given an intravenous infusion of the local

anesthetic lignocaine, which reduces the likelihood of extra electrical activity of the heart (see Intravenous Infusion; Local Anesthetics).

Much can also be done in coronary care units to reduce the risk of VF after a heart attack. Since the risk is greatest during the initial 24 to 48 hours after a heart attack, patients usually stay in a coronary care unit until the critical period has passed. Even so, a number of patients still suffer attacks of VF after this time.

VF outside the hospital

Most heart attacks are unexpected, so patients are more likely to suffer from VF before they can reach the safety of a coronary care unit. The critical period is within the first two hours, so it is imperative to get effective treatment to them immediately. Ideally, there should be teams of paramedics available to rush to the spot when someone collapses with VF. Such teams exist in most U.S. cities, and people trained in resuscitation techniques can often help. Some U.S. cities have even considered providing defibrillators in public places for use in an emergency (see Emergencies).

See also: **Coronary arteries and thrombosis; Heart; Heart attack; Heart disease; Open-heart surgery**

Verruca

My brother is a medical student, and he says that the word "verruca" means any kind of wart, anywhere on the skin. Is this true?

Yes, it is. "Verruca" is the medical term for a wart and doesn't specify the site or appearance. Verruca plantaris, or plantar wart, is a wart on the sole of the foot. People outside the medical profession have shortened the phrase to "verruca," hence the common error. Medical dictionaries have up to a dozen different verruca terms referring to location and shape.

My 13-year-old daughter has a verruca on her sole. Is her younger brother likely to catch it?

Yes. At his age he probably has no immunity to the virus, and so is at risk of being infected. To prevent this, treat your daughter's verruca daily with one of the over-the-counter wart ointments, then cover it with a waterproof adhesive bandage; this will keep her from shedding the virus around the house. Also, she and her brother should use their own towels and footwear, and dry their feet immediately after bathing.

Do preparations bought over the counter really help treat verrucas?

Yes, they do, and in two ways. First, daily application of a wart ointment and rubbing down the horny cap with a pumice stone or emery board will rapidly relieve the pain of walking on a plantar wart. Second, treatment kills the surface virus, thereby reducing the risk of spreading it to others. About 50 percent of plantar warts respond to such simple measures. The treatment must be continued until the wart has completely gone, which usually takes about three months. However, the sufferer often gets discouraged, and so doesn't persist with the treatment for long enough.

Many people know how painful a verruca on the sole of the foot can be, and how persistent. However, it can usually be cured, and very often simply by the sufferer's sheer perseverance with a simple treatment.

The word "verruca" is simply the Latin word for a wart, but is commonly and mistakenly used to mean a wart on the sole of the foot, also known as a plantar wart (the word "plantar" means "on the sole of the foot"). Doctors are consulted more often about these plantar warts than other verrucas because they are more painful and annoying than verrucas elsewhere on the body.

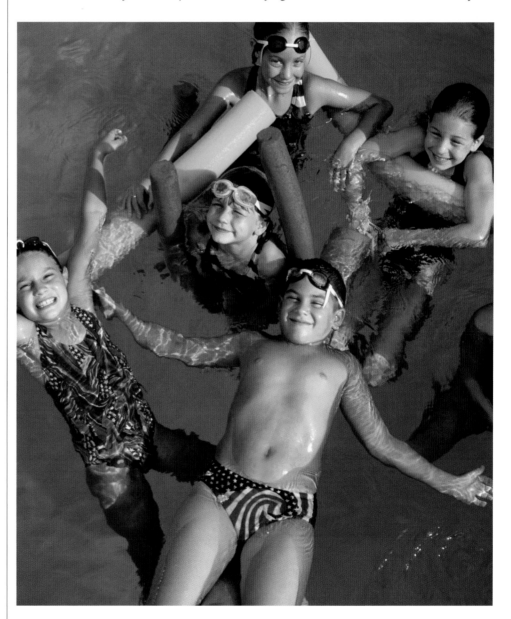

▲ *The verruca plantaris virus is easily spread if the conditions are right. It is particularly prevalent among children, especially when their feet are wet. Keep a plantar wart covered and dry, and make sure that children's feet are thoroughly dried after swimming or bathing. A public pool is often a source of infection, so anyone with a plantar wart should wear plastic or rubber beach shoes.*

Cause

Verrucas are caused by a virus that enters the skin through tiny injuries, especially if the skin is wet and soggy. Most plantar warts arise on the weight-bearing parts of the sole of the foot: that is, the heel and ball, not the instep (see Feet).

A virus is a particle of living matter that can reproduce itself only inside a living cell, borrowing some of the cell's contents for this purpose (see Viruses). After the virus enters the epidermal cell there is an incubation period of several months, while the virus is multiplying and spreading, before enough skin cells are infected and deformed to produce a visible wart.

The epidermal cells deformed by the virus cause a hard, horny swelling (the wart), which on the sole of the foot is pressed inward by standing and walking, thereby irritating the sensitive nerve endings under the skin.

There are several strains of human wart virus. Most plantar warts are caused by the same strain that causes warts elsewhere. Another strain that affects only the soles of the feet causes a mosaic plantar wart. This looks like a honeycomb, and is actually a mass of closely packed polygonal warts, often at least 1 inch (2.5 cm) across. Mosaic plantar warts are extremely resistant to treatment and often last for about 100 years, but are not nearly as painful as common plantar warts.

Verruca plantaris, like other common virus diseases, is unusual in infancy but begins to occur during the school years, reaching a peak at about age nine. It then declines in frequency, becoming rarer after the mid-twenties. Curiously, the sex incidence is equal up to the age of six, but then it becomes more common in girls.

Appearance

Plantar warts are gray or brown with a center of one or more dark pinpoints. The warts are usually rough, bumpy, and spongy, although some may be thick and scaly.

Like plantar warts, corns are also painful, are callous, and appear on the feet, so it may be difficult to tell them apart. However, if the horny cap of a plantar wart is pared away, four distinguishing features will be clearly seen.

First, the wart becomes wider the more skin is pared away. It is shaped like a pyramid with the point at the surface and there is more hidden in the skin than is visible above it. It also has a calloused collar, which pushes aside the tiny lines on the skin of the sole. These never run across the wart but encircle it and its collar. Finally, when the skin can no longer be pared without causing pain, pinpoint bleeding spots appear. If the wart has already been killed, however, the tiny blood vessels are clotted, showing as a few speckled black spots on the surface. This is therefore a sign that the wart is healing.

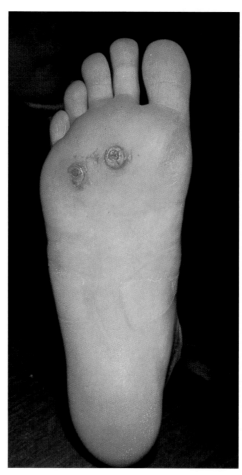

▲ *Plantar warts are particularly painful because they are pressed into the sole of the foot by standing and walking. The calloused skin of each plantar wart should be rubbed down daily, and an over-the-counter wart paint applied.*

In contrast, a corn is widest at the top and narrows to a point within the skin. On paring, it shows a white, smooth appearance like ground glass, and it has no collar. A callus is simply thick skin with a greatly increased epidermal layer. The fine skin lines run through it and are often more obvious in the thick skin of a callus.

Plantar warts occur where the sole touches the ground but—unlike corns and calluses—rarely at an exact point of pressure. Therefore, if the bit of hard painful skin has been present less than two years in a child or young adult, and is not exactly over a bony knot, it is probably a plantar wart. If it has been present more than two years over a bony knob in an older person, it is probably a corn or a callus. Occasionally, a verruca may arise in a callus, and will be revealed by careful paring.

Progress

The verruca plantaris virus, which is relatively harmless and affects only a tiny area of the outer layer of skin, is often overlooked by the body's defenses for many months. This is why plantar warts last so long. Other viruses, like the chicken pox virus (see Chicken Pox), spread throughout the body and rapidly stimulate its chemicals and cellular defenses, so that the illness clears in a week or two. Plantar warts, on the other hand, can last for months or even years.

When the body finally notices the verruca plantaris virus and mounts an offensive, the warts shrivel up and disappear leaving no scar. About 20 percent of plantar warts clear in six months and the majority within two years. Once this immunity is acquired it is readily available to prevent reinfection. Sometimes, as a result of illness or the use of immunosuppressive drugs, this immunity fades and plantar warts recur, so that further treatment will be needed (see Immunosuppressive Drugs).

Treatment

There are no medicines or injections to kill the verruca plantaris virus in the way that antibiotics kill bacteria (see Antibiotics). The aims of local treatment are to destroy the skin cells containing the virus, and to stimulate the body's own defense mechanisms. It is thought that by killing the cells and the virus inside them, the body's defense mechanisms are more readily stimulated. Moreover, local treatment that kills the surface virus makes the plantar warts less infectious to others (see Infection and Infectious Diseases).

Local treatments that can be safely used in the home include ointments, gels, and soaks that contain salicylic acid (a drug that loosens and removes the tough outer layer of skin), lactic acid, formaldehyde, or related drugs. These treatments are applied directly to the skin on on a daily basis, and cause the skin in and

Treating a plantar wart

Wash the foot in warm water, soaking it for at least five minutes.
Dry with a towel (make sure that no one else uses the towel).
Rub the hard skin away with an emery board or pumice stone.
Apply ointment to the plantar wart and let it dry.
Cover with an adhesive bandage.
Have your nurse or doctor check the plantar wart each month.
Continue treatment daily until the nurse or doctor thinks it is cured.
See your doctor if the plantar wart becomes more painful.

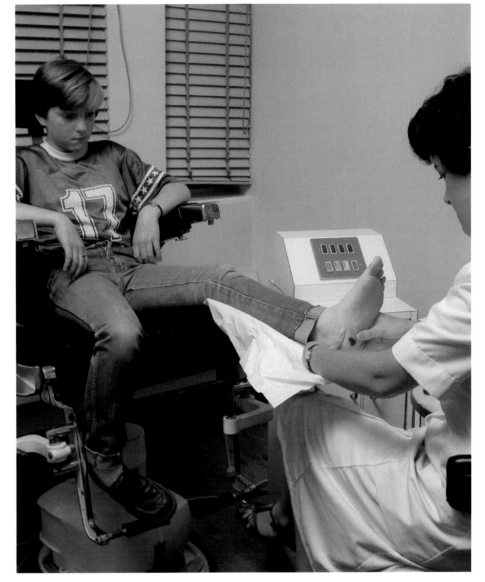

around the plantar wart to gradually disintegrate. Rubbing down the calloused cap of a plantar wart relieves the pain of walking on it, and if this is not done, a layer of dead, hard tissue builds up over the wart, shielding it from the ointment that has to be put on.

If there are many small plantar warts, an alternative treatment is to soak the affected sole in a saucer of formalin in solution every night and morning for 10 minutes. Since formalin dries out the skin, causing it to crack, the skin between the toes and around the wart should be protected with petroleum jelly.

Salicylic acid can be used in the form of plasters, although stronger preparations, such as Chlorsal and Posalfilin, can cause inflammation in normal skin and should be used only under medical supervision.

Any treatment may take up to three months. It is easy to tell if a plantar wart is cured, because it ceases to hurt. Tiny black spots can be seen in it, and the skin then returns to normal.

If the verruca plantaris persists, the next step is treatment by freezing with liquid nitrogen, known as cryotherapy, which has to be given by a doctor or at a hospital. The wart will turn black and fall off within a few days, although sometimes the cold may not penetrate enough to kill the virus completely. If this treatment is unavailable, the core of the wart can be scooped out under local anesthesia, and the base and sides cauterized (see Local Anesthetics). The resulting hole is covered with a sterile dressing, and kept dry until it heals (see Dressings and Bandages). Plantar warts are never cut out, since this would leave a scar that might be persistently painful.

▲ *The key to curing a verruca plantaris is persistence, since some can take months to disappear. The progress of the plantar wart should be checked every month by a doctor, a nurse, or podiatrist, who will be able to tell when it has healed completely and, therefore, when continual treatment is no longer necessary.*

The most modern, clean, accurate, and effective treatment for plantar warts is laser surgery. However, because this is also the most expensive treatment, some doctors do not offer it, so other treatments are usually tried first.

Prevention

Most plantar warts are caught at swimming pools. This is because the skin barrier is weaker when it is wet. People with plantar warts should therefore wear thin rubber or plastic beach shoes.

In the home, a child can be prevented from spreading the virus by using his or her own towel and bath mat, and by covering the plantar wart with a waterproof adhesive plaster.

See also: **Corns; Hygiene; Podiatry; Skin and skin diseases; Warts**

Vertigo

Questions and Answers

I often feel dizzy when I stand up suddenly, especially after having a hot bath. Is this vertigo?

No. This is postural hypotension, in which the blood pressure drops slightly but suddenly so that the blood supply to the brain is reduced a little. It happens to everyone occasionally and does not usually signify anything serious, unless it happens often, in which case you should see your doctor.

Some years ago my father had a serious heart infection and he has suffered from vertigo ever since. Could this be due to his treatment?

There are some antibiotics that can cause vertigo as a side effect, though this is an uncommon reaction, and your father may have needed these drugs when he was ill. These antibiotics can damage the inner ear's balance receptors, so their use is reserved purely for life-threatening situations.

How do trapeze artists avoid vertigo, which would be dangerous when they work so high in the air?

Such people avoid getting vertigo by practicing. They are trained to ignore the violent stimulation of their balance sensors, which would otherwise cause vertigo. The artists perform regular exercises that gradually enable them to prevent vertigo. Similar exercises can help some people who suffer from vertigo for medical reasons.

Why do some people get vertigo when they are looking down from great heights?

People who are afraid of heights usually feel faintness rather than true vertigo. Vertigo refers to a feeling that the world is spinning around you, or that you are moving or swaying when you are really standing still.

People often confuse vertigo with a fear of heights. In fact, it can be a symptom of a variety of conditions, from the normal effects of spinning on a merry-go-round to the distressing results of some sort of brain damage.

Vertigo is a common and often distressing symptom that occurs when the delicate balance mechanisms in the inner part of the ear or brain stem are damaged or disturbed. Many of the causes of vertigo are not at all serious, but sometimes vertigo can indicate a dangerous disease.

The balance mechanism
The position of the head is continuously monitored by sensitive mechanisms in the inner ear, which act like levels. When the head is moved, the fluid inside the inner ear's balance center is set in motion. As this fluid moves, it stimulates tiny hairs that are connected to nerve fibers. These nerve fibers inform the brain of the head's rotary motion. If the movement stops suddenly, the fluid continues to move and the brain continues to get messages that the head is still turning.

Information from the inner ear is sent to the brain stem, the area of the brain responsible for interpreting information from the balance centers. However, the brain stem also receives information about the body's position from the eyes and other position sensors. These other sensors tell the brain that the movement has stopped. This contradictory information confuses the brain, which is receiving false and incoherent messages. A picture of an unstable and chaotic world is formed in the brain stem and this results in vertigo (see Brain).

This common type of vertigo can be cured very simply by spinning a little in the opposite direction. This sets the fluid sensors in contrary motion to counteract the first spin. Ballet

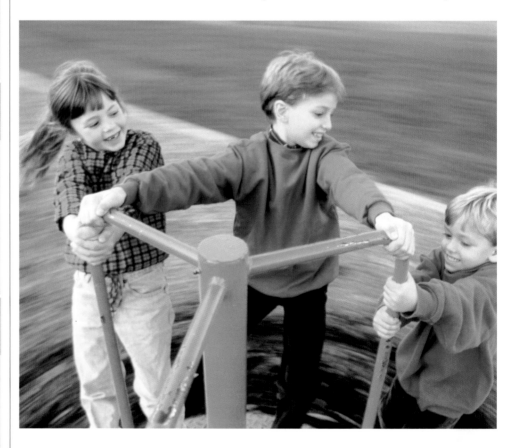

▲ *Children love merry-go-rounds such as this one because spinning around and around makes them delightfully dizzy. They relish such deliberate episodes of vertigo.*

dancers and circus performers, who have to spin violently during their routines, can train themselves not to suffer from vertigo.

Medically, vertigo can be caused in two ways: there can be something wrong with the inner ear mechanism so that the messages get confused, or the brain stem itself can be damaged so that messages are not properly analyzed.

Problems in the inner ear

The part of the inner ear that contains the balance sensors is called the labyrinth, because it curls into a spiral. The labyrinth can sometimes be the site of a viral infection, which can cause sudden and severe vertigo, called labyrinthitis (see Viruses). Sometimes the sensation of spinning is so strong that it causes vomiting, and even slight head movements can cause dizziness (see Vomiting).

This condition is called positional vertigo and the symptoms may continue during convalescence. Drugs that sedate the balance centers in the brain stem can be a very effective treatment for the unpleasant spinning sensation.

Persistent positional vertigo is caused by tiny specks of hard material that are a by-product of the infection in the labyrinth. These tiny specks of material or stones lie near the tiny hairs within the inner ear, rolling onto these sensory hairs whenever the head moves. As they do so they stimulate the nerve endings and tell the brain that the head is spinning when information received from all the other sensors says that the body is still.

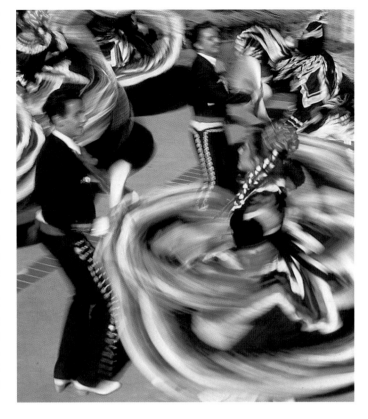

▼ *Peering up into the Manhattan skyline can bring on dizziness: the confused brain wants to believe that the buildings rather than the clouds are moving.*

▲ *Flamenco dancers avoid spinning themselves dizzy by spotting: they focus their eyes on one spot for as long as possible and come back to the same spot each time around.*

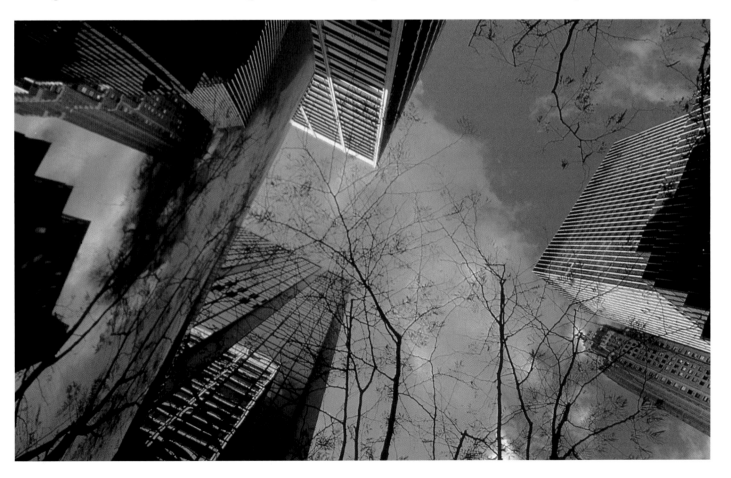

Labyrinthitis can be caused as a result of a flulike illness (see Influenza) or as a result of other types of ear infection, such as otitis media. This type of ear infection is common among children. However, vertigo is a rare complication of this condition (see Otitis).

Ménière's disease can also cause vertigo. It happens when there is a rise of pressure in the fluid cavities of the inner ear, including the balance mechanisms. It is not known exactly why this happens, but it is usually characterized by severe vertigo with partial loss of hearing and a continuous buzzing in the affected ear. The buzzing is called tinnitus.

The symptoms of vertigo can be treated with special drugs. However, the partial deafness is sometimes permanent, and Ménière's disease is one of the causes of vertigo that require the sufferer to seek prompt medical advice (see Deafness).

Damage to the brain stem

Nerve messages from the inner ear are analyzed by the cerebellum and by a collection of cells in the brain stem called the vestibular nucleus. Damage to this interpretative part of the system can also cause vertigo (see Brain Damage and Disease).

In older people, the blood vessels that supply the brain stem can become furred or even blocked. Starved of sufficient oxygen, cells in the brain stem stop working and messages from the inner ear are no longer properly analyzed.

Sometimes the blood vessels get kinked in the neck as a result of arthritic neck joints (see Arthritis). As a result, the blood supply may be momentarily blocked when the head is turned suddenly. This can produce vertigo. Occasionally, tumors or patches of inflammation may affect the vestibular nucleus, producing vertigo (see Inflammation).

All these types of vertigo can be eased by drugs, but the root cause also has to be found and treated by a doctor. Vertigo can also be a symptom of a stroke or of multiple sclerosis (see Multiple Sclerosis).

Vertigo caused by drugs

There are many drugs that cause vertigo, perhaps the most common being alcohol. Large quantities of alcohol can make the world appear very unsteady indeed, especially when a person is lying down with closed eyes (see Alcoholism). Closing the eyes is likely to bring on sudden, mild vertigo because the eyes provide information that can contradict the confused messages coming from the balance centers in the inner ear.

HOW VERTIGO OCCURS

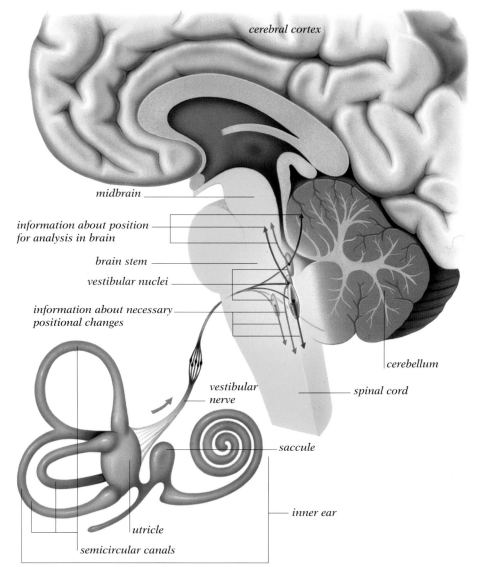

cerebral cortex

midbrain

information about position for analysis in brain

brain stem

vestibular nuclei

information about necessary positional changes

cerebellum

spinal cord

vestibular nerve

saccule

inner ear

utricle

semicircular canals

▲ *Vertigo can be brought on by two different sets of conditions: either confused messages are sent to the brain from the semicircular canals in the ears, or some damage to the vestibular nucleus causes the messages that are received to be incorrectly analyzed.*

Outlook

It has recently been shown that many cases of benign positional vertigo, a common affliction of older people, can be cured by a definite sequence of movements of the head to rotate the rear semicircular canal so that a plug of debris is displaced into the urticle where it has no effect. This is called the Epley maneuver, and it may have to be repeated from time to time.

Persistent or regular vertigo should always prompt a visit to the doctor so that it can be investigated. Provided this is done, the outlook is generally very good.

The ability of the brain to unscramble confused messages is remarkable. Most forms of vertigo will actually disappear in time, because the brain eventually learns to interpret the conflicting messages and to ignore those that are false.

See also: **Balance; Dizziness; Ménière's disease; Nervous system; Tinnitus**

Virginity

I am 21 years old and a virgin. My partner wants to sleep with me, but I am afraid that losing my virginity will hurt. Are my fears well-founded?

The first time can be painful for some people, both men and women. If the woman's hymen is intact, she may experience some pain when it is ruptured. In most women, however, tampons and sports activities will have stretched the hymen to the point where the bleeding and pain will be slight. It is more likely that any pain you might feel will be caused by fear and nervousness, making you tense and likely to have insufficient lubrication in your vagina. Take it slowly, and make sure that both you and your partner are aroused and comfortable; you will find that the pleasure will soon outweigh any pain you felt the first time.

My boyfriend says that I don't love him because I don't want to go beyond heavy petting. What can I say to him?

You could equally claim that he doesn't love you because he wants to force or persuade you to do something you don't wish to do. Sex never proved anything, certainly not love. People have sex for many reasons, and too often out of the misguided conviction that it is expected of them. Don't fall into this trap: if you do not want to make love, then that is your right, and your boyfriend should respect your decision. Wait until you feel it is the right time.

I'm about to go to college and I'm still a virgin. Is this at all unusual?

It is true that by the age of 19 virgins are in the minority, and about 75 percent of your colleagues will have lost their virginity. However, it's nothing to be ashamed of. The choice of how you run your sex life is your own.

All aspects of sexual behavior can provoke the deepest of emotional reactions in people. Nowhere is this more true than over the issue of virginity—or, more precisely, its loss.

A virgin is simply someone who has never had sexual intercourse. There is a tendency for people to think of women when the word "virgin" is mentioned, but in fact the word actually applies to both sexes equally. The word "virgin" derives from the ancient Greek word *virgo*, meaning "maiden," but the term "virgin" has been used since the year 1300 to apply to men as well as women. Rather unfairly, however, the stigma attached to women who lose their virginity outside marriage has generally been greater than for the male sex. Medically speaking, virginity is a physical state and a person cannot be "almost" a virgin. A person either has or hasn't had sexual intercourse. Since there is one physical change that can occur to a woman on her first experience of sex, this is seen by many people and cultures as proof of virginity (see Sex).

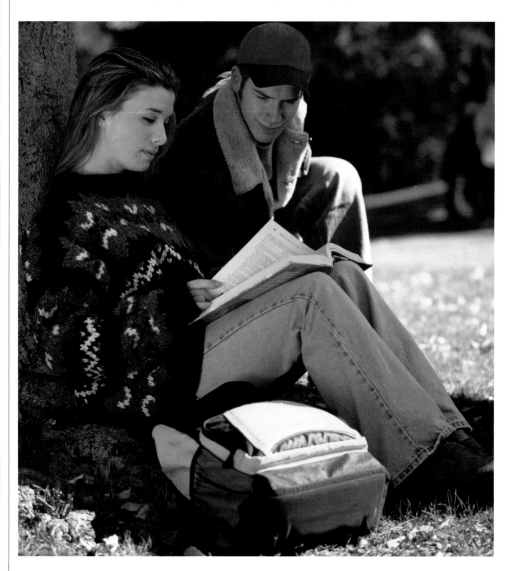

▲ *Adolescence is a time of rapid change, especially in attitudes toward the opposite sex. It is important that young people take on their adult roles at their own pace and do not allow themselves to be pressured into premature sexual activity.*

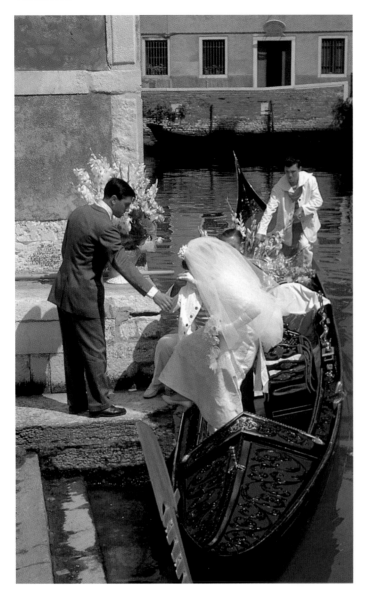

▲ *Catholicism places a high value on a woman's virginity on her wedding day. A bride disembarks in Venice dressed in white as a symbol of her virginity. Catholic women are taught to imitate the Virgin Mary, who epitomizes purity and grace and the sanctity of the body.*

The hymen

The majority of virgin women have a thin membrane that partially closes off the vagina. This is called the hymen. It can be very thin or fairly tough; it can close off the vagina almost completely, leaving only a small opening for the monthly period, or be so flimsy as to be no barrier at all (see Vagina).

The hymen can be stretched or broken over the years by virgins who have used tampons for their periods, masturbated, or even engaged energetically in some sports (see Masturbation). The hymen can also be stretched or broken during heavy petting. However, none of these conditions is a loss of virginity.

Conversely, a hymen can be tough enough to resist complete penetration by the man and, in some cases, will stretch but not break. There have been cases of virgin births, with women giving birth although the hymen was still intact.

In most cases, the thin membrane will be in place and will break the first time the woman has intercourse. This may cause bleeding and pain in some women. On subsequent occasions, the ring of tissue will wear away until it becomes virtually nonexistent. However, the lack of a hymen, or lack of pain and bleeding, is absolutely no proof that the woman was not a virgin.

Advantages and disadvantages

There are a number of benefits to being a virgin. Virgin women, of course, do not have unwanted pregnancies or catch sexually transmitted diseases (see Sexually Transmitted Diseases). There is also some evidence that nuns are less likely to suffer from cancer of the cervix (see Cervix and Cervical Smears). On the other hand, nuns are more likely to get breast cancer (see Breasts) than women who are sexually active. Cancer of the cervix is linked to the human papilloma virus and thus to the number of sexual partners, whereas breast cancer seems to occur more frequently in women who have not been pregnant (see Cancer). There may also be emotional as well as physical benefits to virginity. If a person has been brought up to believe that it is important to remain a virgin, either until a specific time, like marriage, or for life, then there is a strong chance that he or she will suffer emotionally by giving in to the persuasion of other people.

Many societies place great emphasis on women being virgins on their wedding day. This is probably because in a patriarchal, or male-ruled, society the only way a man could be certain his property and name were being handed on to his son was to make sure his woman did not get pregnant by another man—especially before the wedding. In such societies, visible proof of virginity may even be demanded, and bloodstained bedsheets have to be displayed after the wedding night. Indeed, some Italian gynecologists do a flourishing trade in surgically restoring hymens for such an occasion (see Gynecology).

Defloration

Losing one's virginity is something that should happen happily, leaving no feelings of fear, guilt, or self-disgust. In fact, it is hardly something a person should lose, but something that should be given and shared with someone that he or she loves. The first time a person makes love is very important, less for the mere tearing of a membrane than for the psychological impact invested in the occasion. Virginity is also a state of mind, and a 30-year-old mother can be virginal in her approach to life, while a 14-year-old may be tough, cynical, and far from innocent even though he or she has never had sex. The most important thing that a person should consider about giving up his or her virginity is being sure that it is being done at the time that is right for him or her. Nobody should lose his or her virginity (or, indeed, ever have sex at any time in life) simply because "Everybody's doing it," or because someone says, "Honestly, you're not still a virgin at your age."

There are no firm rules about when men or women should lose their virginity. As with all good things, waiting, anticipating, and planning can enhance the event, so leaping into bed with the first partner, or as soon after the 16th birthday as possible, is hardly a good idea. The right time is when it feels right.

See also: **Abstinence; Adolescence; Hymen; Intercourse**

Viruses

Why is it that viruses cannot be treated with antibiotics?

Bacteria that respond to antibiotics are complicated organisms, although each consists of only one cell. Viruses, on the other hand, are very simple, consisting of a core of nucleic acid (genetic material) surrounded by a protein capsule. Antibiotics work by impeding the activity of the bacterial cell without harming human cells. However, virus metabolism and structure are quite different from those of bacteria, so antibiotics that attack bacterial structure and metabolism have no effect on viruses.

Is it likely that any new treatments will be able to affect the course of minor viral diseases like the common cold?

It seems unlikely that any form of direct treatment for minor viral diseases will be discovered in the near future, unless a sudden major breakthrough in the research of viruses occurs.

It has been very difficult to make a vaccine against the common cold because the common cold is caused by some 200 viruses and these viruses are always mutating. The natural antiviral substances in the interferon range of drugs do have some useful effects against viruses, but the high expense of producing these drugs makes them impractical for general use. However, there are nearly 20 different antiviral drugs currently in use—most of them acting to inhibit the synthesis of DNA or RNA in the viruses, or to inhibit viral uncoating—and the range of antiviral drugs is continually growing. Therefore, it seems likely that, eventually, effective treatments may be found for many minor viral infections. In the meantime, the best approach to minor viral diseases may be in prevention rather than cure.

Influenza, measles, and rabies are disparate diseases that have something in common: being caused by viruses. An increasing number of diseases caused by viruses can now be effectively treated by new antiviral drugs, and new drugs are constantly being developed.

The work of great people like Louis Pasteur (1822–1895) led to the discovery of bacteria—the cause of many of the most serious illnesses. However, by the end of the 19th century there were still many diseases for which a bacterial cause was suspected but not found. Pasteur had demonstrated that rabies was an infection and had produced a vaccine against it, but he had not been able to find a bacterium that caused it. He rightly deduced that this was because the organism was too small to be seen under a microscope.

The first virus was found in 1892 and was identified as tobacco mosaic virus. This virus causes disease in plants rather than in humans. Following this discovery it was shown that

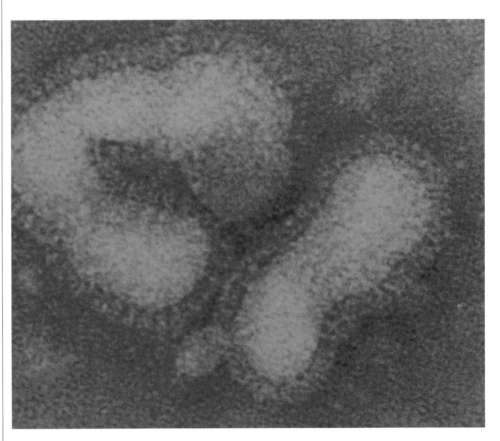

▲ *Viruses are extremely simple structures that usually consist of a thin protein membrane containing one of the nucleic acids, DNA or RNA. The influenza virus (above) is a typical example. It is also wrapped in an outer envelope, as shown in the model (top). The influenza virus can change its protein structure with each new infection in order to fool the body's immune system.*

HOW A VIRUS MULTIPLIES

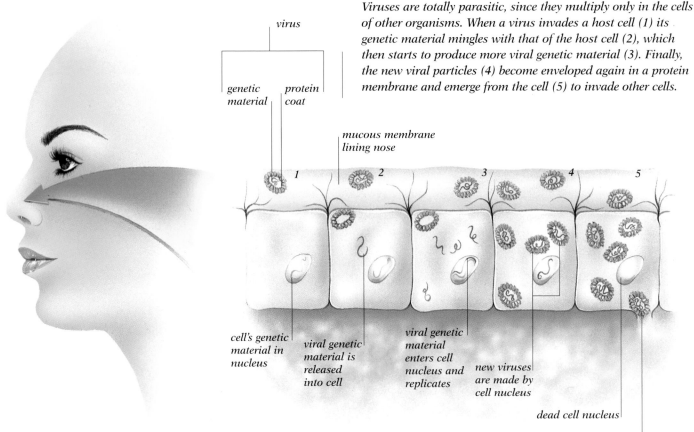

Viruses are totally parasitic, since they multiply only in the cells of other organisms. When a virus invades a host cell (1) its genetic material mingles with that of the host cell (2), which then starts to produce more viral genetic material (3). Finally, the new viral particles (4) become enveloped again in a protein membrane and emerge from the cell (5) to invade other cells.

virus

genetic material   protein coat

mucous membrane lining nose

1   2   3   4   5

cell's genetic material in nucleus

viral genetic material is released into cell

viral genetic material enters cell nucleus and replicates

new viruses are made by cell nucleus

dead cell nucleus

cell ruptures releasing viruses

▼ *The hepatitis A virus is often found in bad food and water. The infection thus occurs in areas with poor sanitation.*

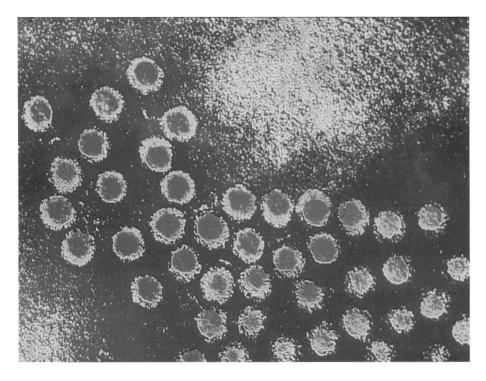

foot-and-mouth disease, which occurs in cattle, was caused by a similar tiny organism.

It was demonstrated that these viruses were able to travel from plant to plant or animal to animal after passing through a filter too fine to let a bacterium through.

Research was carried out in the light of knowledge at the time, but was impeded by the fact that it was still not possible to see viruses. It was the electron microscope that first revealed what viruses actually look like.

What are viruses?

Viruses are very tiny organisms. For example, a polio virus is 20 nanometers across (a nanometer is one-thousandth of a micrometer, which in turn is one-thousandth of a millimeter; see Poliomyelitis).

The basic structure of viruses is so simple that it is questionable whether they should be regarded as living matter at all. Essentially, they consist of no more than a capsule of protein that contains their genetic material in the form of one of the nucleic acids, DNA or RNA (see Protein).

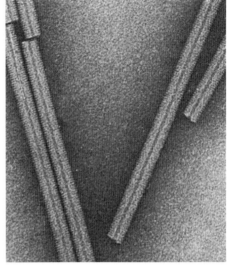

▲ *The first virus to be discovered was the tobacco mosaic virus. It is viewed here under the electron microscope, which enabled research to progress.*

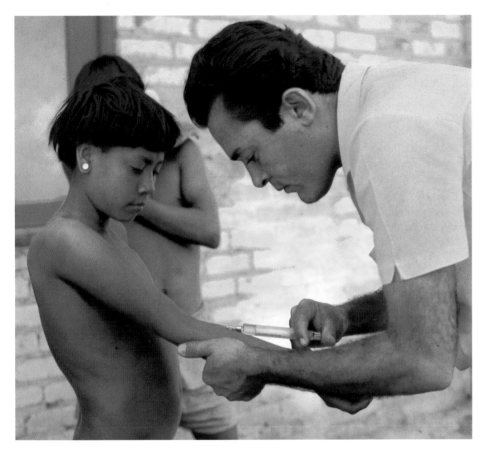

◄ *Vaccination is vital for preventing the deadliest viral infections, especially in developing countries where so many other serious health problems are rife.*

These are the substances that carry the genetic message from generation to generation in all living things (see Genetics). It is the DNA that is passed on in the process of reproduction and is contained in the nucleus of living cells. The DNA then sends messages to the chemical factories inside the cells, instructing them to make various types of protein. These messages are carried by the RNA.

Viruses work by invading the cells of the organism they are infecting. Once a virus is inside a cell, it inserts its DNA into the DNA of the cell, and the protein-producing apparatus of the cell starts to work for the virus instead of for the cell itself. Having taken control of a cell, the virus manufactures more viruses, so that more cells and finally other individuals can be infected (see Cells and Chromosomes).

Therefore, viruses are very lifelike in their ability to pass on their own characteristics from generation to generation by the use of genetic material. The two nucleic acids, DNA and RNA, are the basic stuff of life, and even if they are contained in only a thin capsule, they make up what is virtually a living organism.

Structure

Viruses are extremely small, the smallest being 20–30 nanometers across and the largest 10 times that size. Most viruses are more or less round in shape. Exceptions are the rabies virus and its related viruses, which are bullet-shaped; and the smallpox virus and its related viruses, which are brick-shaped (see Smallpox).

Viruses are basically classified according to whether they carry the nucleic acid DNA or RNA. The nucleic acid core of a virus is called the genome and the protein capsule the capsid. The capsid is made up from many identical protein blocks called capsomeres. The way in which the capsomeres line up around the genome dictates the overall shape of the individual virus particle.

Different groups of viruses have different shapes, one of the most common being the icosahedron, a structure with 20 flat sides of equal size, effectively forming a sphere. The capsid of other viruses forms a hollow cylinder. These differences in structure can be determined only by pictures taken with an electron microscope (electron micrographs). Some viruses have another structure on top of their capsid, aptly called an envelope.

All these variations place a virus in a particular group. The viruses that cause human disease are now all classified. The five hepatitis B viruses are classified as hepadnaviruses (hepatitis DNA viruses), and the hepatitis A virus is classified as a picornavirus (pico RNA virus); "pico" means "very small."

Viruses and bacteria

There is an enormous difference in size between viruses and bacteria. For example, a streptococcus is 50 times greater in diameter than a polio virus (see Bacteria; Streptococcus).

An individual bacterium is able to reproduce itself by splitting in two, and it can live independently, having the apparatus to carry out many metabolic processes within its cell wall (see Metabolism). All bacteria contain DNA and RNA. In contrast, although viruses can survive outside the cells of other organisms, they need these cells to supply them with building materials and enable them to reproduce. They do this by making exact copies of themselves according to instructions from their DNA or RNA, a process known as replication. They contain only one kind of nucleic acid.

How are viruses spread?

Viral diseases can be very infectious. A disease like measles is so infectious that until vaccination was introduced, it was certain that virtually every child in the United States would get it. A new epidemic used to occur about every two years.

The measles virus, like many others, is spread by droplet infection. A cough or sneeze from an infected person will carry the virus into the air to be inhaled by someone else (see Measles).

The polio virus and enteroviruses (primarily infecting the intestines) enter the body via the digestive tract. Another group, the togaviruses, which are carried by insects, make their way into the body through the skin as the result of an insect bite. Rabies also enters via a bite from an animal that has been driven to distraction by the disease.

The rhinoviruses that are responsible for the common cold enter the cells of the mucous membrane joining the nose to create symptoms in the nose and upper airways (see Membranes; Mucus).

Once inside the body, viruses invade the cells, usually selecting one particular type of body cell.

Viruses in the laboratory

Viruses not only are difficult to see but are very difficult to grow in the laboratory, since they depend on living cells for replication. In the early days of virology it was not possible to grow viruses at all; it was possible only to pass them from one laboratory animal to another.

The first advances in this field came with the realization that viruses could be grown inside fertilized chickens' eggs. The influenza, mumps, and herpes viruses can all be grown in this way by injecting infected tissue into the inside of the egg. This will produce a collection of tiny colonies just like those on a bacterial culture plate.

The next step was the development of tissue cultures, which are collections of mammalian cells grown in a test tube. Preparing a culture is not a routine technique of investigation, but it is vitally important in the making of vaccines that protect us against the most dangerous and widespread viral infections.

A particular viral infection is usually diagnosed by monitoring the levels of antibodies in a patient's blood over a period of two weeks.

Treatment of viral infections

The AIDS pandemic has resulted in an enormous expansion in research into viruses and the details of their life cycles and modes of reproduction. As new facts were discovered, it became possible to produce new drugs that interfered with various aspects of these reproductive processes. As a result, some 20 antiviral drugs are now in general use. Diseases against which these agents are effective include AIDS, influenza A and B, herpes simplex infections, cytomegalovirus infections, hepatitis B and C, and Lassa fever. Combinations of antiviral drugs can reduce HIV replications to levels undetectable in the circulation and postpone the development of AIDS.

Antiviral drugs work in several different ways. Some replace substances that viruses build into their structure. Some replace chemicals that viruses need to produce the enzymes necessary for DNA replication (DNA polymerases). Some act to block the processes of virus uncoating so that the genome cannot be released. Antiretroviral agents, such as those used to kill HIV, act by inhibiting the viral enzyme (reverse transcriptase) that catalyzes the conversion of RNA into DNA. HIV protease inhibitor drugs block another essential viral enzyme (see Enzymes).

Prevention

Many serious viral infections can be prevented. Smallpox was eradicated worldwide through a combination of vaccination and

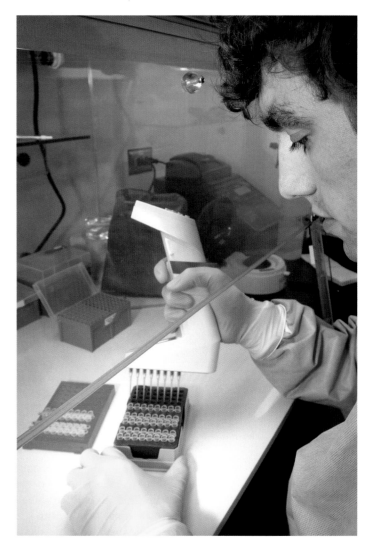

▲ *SARS virus tests are being done at the Viral and Rickettsial Diseases Division of Centers for Disease Control and Prevention.*

isolation of cases. Vaccinations also exist for measles, rubella (German measles), yellow fever, polio, and rabies (see Rubella; Yellow Fever).

There are some infections, however, against which it is more difficult to produce an effective vaccine. New viruses, such as SARS, need to be thoroughly studied before a vaccine can be attempted (see SARS). Other viruses, such as influenza, have a remarkable ability to change their protein structure as they pass from person to person. These minor changes enable them to fool the body's immune system with each new infection. This explains why people get so many attacks of the same disease in a lifetime.

A vaccine will be effective if it is made from the current strain of a virus, but for this to be possible, a manufacturer would have to predict the strain accurately, which would be a very difficult proposition. The problem is multiplied in the case of the common cold, since it involves so many viral strains. Therefore, it is unlikely that prevention or treatments for the common cold will be available in the near future.

See also: AIDS; Common cold; Hepatitis; Herpes; Immune system; Infection and infectious diseases; Influenza; Measles; Rabies; Vaccinations

Vitamin A

Questions and Answers

If halibut-liver oil is good for me, is a double dose twice as good?

Halibut-liver oil is a valuable source of vitamin A, but it is dangerous to exceed the recommended dose. Because vitamin A is stored in the body, excessive amounts can be toxic.

Does vitamin A prevent colds?

Vitamin A aids the body in producing mucus-secreting cells, and In this way the body protects itself from germs. It works by removing them from the body—by the nose in the case of a cold. A lack of vitamin A makes you more likely to catch colds.

Is it true that eating carrots will help me see in the dark?

There is no truth in this old wives' tale. Visual purple in the light-sensitive retinal cells needs vitamin A, but you would have to be severely deficient for its function to be affected. Taking more will not improve vision.

Is a poor diet the only cause of vitamin A deficiency?

No, not in developed countries. The usual cause is the failure of the intestine to absorb enough vitamin A, which may be due to malabsorption syndromes or other damage to the intestine. Deficiency can occur as a side effect of long-term treatment with anticholesterol drugs. Diets with low levels of fat and retinol can also cause a deficiency.

What are the symptoms of vitamin A deficiency?

A deficiency results in night blindness. The eyes become dry and inflamed, with eventual corneal damage.

Deficiency in vitamin A is relatively rare in the West, but when it does occur, generally owing to malabsorption, serious health problems are the result, including eventual blindness.

Vitamin A is one of the vital groups of vitamins that the body needs to function properly. It enables people to see in a dim light, keeps the skin healthy, ensures normal growth, and renews the body tissue. With only a few exceptions, all the necessary vitamins are obtained from food, and the minute amounts the body requires mostly exist in their natural state in food. Vitamin A, however, is largely manufactured by the body from a food substance called carotene.

Sources of vitamin A

The vitamin A in food comes in two different forms from two different sources. The pure form, called retinol, is found in foods such as fish liver oils, liver, kidney, cheese, eggs, and butter, and has already been manufactured by the animal concerned. The second form is made in the body from carotene, which is found in such vegetables as carrots, spinach, cabbage, and tomatoes.

Vegetables are orange, yellow, or dark green in color because of carotene, and the darker the green, the greater the carotene content. Spinach and watercress contain more carotene in each pound than cabbage, and dark green cabbage provides more than lighter-colored vegetables. Carotene is converted into retinol in the liver and in the small intestine, and then some of the vitamin A in the form of converted carotene or retinol is absorbed into the bloodstream and circulated around the body to be used in its everyday functions, while the rest is stored in the liver.

Although vitamin A is not present in many foods, those that contain it are readily available. A fifth of people's average intake comes from vegetables, mainly carrots. Turnips and potatoes are no substitute, however, since they contain no carotene. Milk and butter are other common sources; margarine, to which vitamin A is added artificially, contains almost as much vitamin A as butter and is therefore nutritionally comparable.

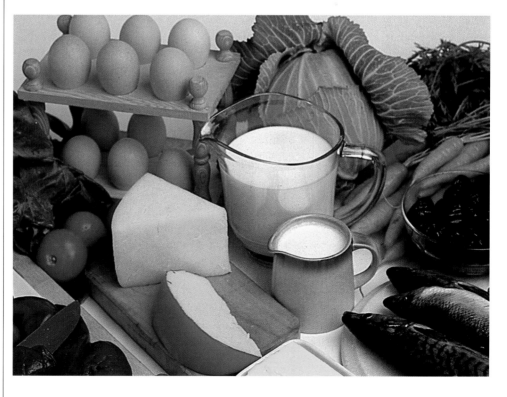

▲ *Dairy products, fish, liver, and certain vegetables contain high levels of Vitamin A.*

Vitamin A: Are you getting enough?

The daily requirement for different age groups and the vitamin A content in the foods listed are given in micrograms (1,000 micrograms = 1 milligram, or one-thousandth of a gram). If someone is unable to take the correct amount every day, it is necessary only for him or her to regulate the amount taken over a week and ensure that it gives the correct daily average.

Age group		Daily requirement
Babies	0–12 months	450
Children:	1–3 years	300
	4–8 years	400
	9–13 years	600
Adolescent and adult men (14+)		900
Adolescent and adult women (14+)		700
Expectant mothers:	14–18 years	750
	19+ years	770
Lactating mothers:	14–18 years	1,200
	19+ years	1,300

Vitamin A content of foods

Food	Vitamin A content
Apricots, dried, 2 oz. (57 g)	340
Butter, 1 oz. (28 g)	282
Cabbage, 4 oz. (114 g)	56
Carrots, 4 oz. (114 g)	2,267
Cheese, 2 oz. (57 g)	238
Cod-liver oil capsule, 1	180
Cream, heavy, 2 tbsp. (30 ml)	130
Egg, 1	80
Halibut-oil capsule, 1	1,200
Kidney, 4 o.z (114 g)	340
Fish, oily, 4 oz. (114 g)	52
Liver, cow, 4 oz. (114 g)	6,800
Margarine, 1 oz. (28 g)	255
Milk, whole, 7 fl. oz. (0.2 L)	80
Peas, frozen, 4 oz. (114 g)	56
Prunes, dried, 2 oz. (57 g)	90
Spinach, 4 oz. (114 g)	1,136
Tomato, 1½ oz. (42 g)	49
Watercress, 1 oz. (28 g)	142

Foods rich in vitamin A tend to retain their vitamin content, although prolonged exposure to light and air can reduce the amount. Cooking at normal temperatures has no serious effect, but frying at a high temperature will result in loss of vitamin content.

Vitamin A deficiency

A lack of vitamin A can cause itching, burning, and reddened eyelids, and a drastic deficiency can lead to blindness. Many children in developing countries are vulnerable as a result of early weaning onto an unsuitable food like skim milk, which contains little or no vitamin A. However, prepared baby foods usually have essential vitamins added to them. In more affluent societies the diet tends to be better balanced, and most people get as much vitamin A as they need; about two-thirds of it comes from retinol and one-third from carotene. Nevertheless, a deficiency of vitamin A can cause night blindness (see Night Blindness). Normally it takes about seven to 10 minutes for the eyes to become used to a dim light; so if someone cannot distinguish objects in the twilight, vitamin A deficiency may be the reason. Halibut-liver oil capsules can be taken, since this oil is one of the best sources of vitamin A. When people have a high-protein diet, they are at risk of deficiency because the body uses up the vitamin faster when converting protein into body tissue and energy. The body also uses up its store of vitamin A quickly during fevers. Certain drugs can cause a loss; a doctor will advise how much vitamin A is needed in any of these situations.

Because vitamin A is stored in the liver, daily intake is not essential, although regular supplies are needed. Too much vitamin A can be taken from an excess of halibut oil capsules. Symptoms include insomnia, weight loss, dryness of the lips, and aching limbs. Taking slightly more than is needed is unlikely to cause harm.

See also: **Diet; Fevers; Vitamins**

Vitamin B

I'm on the Pill and suffer from headaches and depression. Would a B vitamin supplement be helpful?

Since the Pill is said to result in pyridoxine deficiency, you can try taking more of this vitamin. Start with 2–5 mg a day and increase this if symptoms persist. You can also add brown rice, liver, chicken, mackerel, peanuts, brewer's yeast, and wheat germ to your diet. For a general supplement, take B-complex capsules.

Does drinking too much alcohol cause a vitamin B deficiency?

Yes. Heavy drinking provides enough calories and so reduces food intake, resulting in deficiency of the B vitamins. The poor concentration, fatigue, and weight loss alcoholics suffer from may be due as much to thiamine deficiency as excessive drinking.

Drink less, or if you find it difficult to cut down, make sure your diet contains more milk, whole-meal bread, beef, fortified cereal, and peanuts.

My son will eat only white rice and bread. Could he get beriberi?

This is unlikely. The association of beriberi with white cereals is not due to eating the cereals; it is due to eating virtually nothing else. White rice and white bread are not sources of thiamine. However, while wheat flour (hence whole wheat bread) is supplemented with thiamine by law, most diets contain other sources of thiamine.

Is it possible to take too much vitamin B?

Theoretically no, since the vitamin is not stored in the body and any excess is excreted. However, very large doses might constitute a major challenge to your system, and could have a toxic effect.

Vitamin B is essential for some of the body's biochemical processes. Unlike most other vitamins, it is not stored in the body and needs to be consumed daily. It is present in a wide variety of foods, however, and deficiency is unusual.

Vitamin B is a complex of at least eight separate water-soluble vitamins: B1 (thiamine), B2 (riboflavin), B3 (niacin), folic acid (folacin), B6 (pyridoxine), B12 (cyanocobalamin), biotin, and pantothenic acid. People can obtain the B vitamins in adequate supplies if they eat a well-balanced diet, since these vitamins are present in a wide variety of foods.

Nonetheless, B vitamins can be destroyed easily, and their absorption and use by the body are affected by drugs or excessive consumption of alcohol. If a deficiency occurs, disease can result.

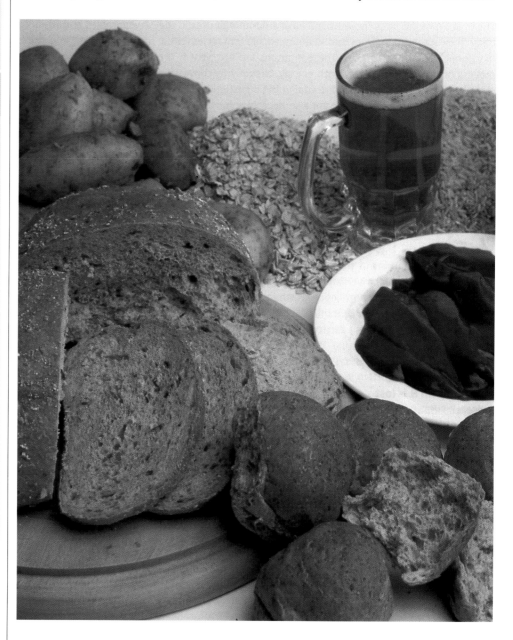

▲ *A good diet is the best guarantee of adequate vitamin B, which is present in a variety of foods such as whole-grain bread and cereals, liver, and root vegetables.*

Vitamin C

My mother says that freezing and canning take all the vitamin C out of vegetables. Is she right?

There may be a slight loss when vegetables are blanched for freezing, and a further slight loss if frozen vegetables are stored for a long time. However, fresh vegetables that have also been stored may yield less vitamin C than frozen ones, since it is readily destroyed by contact with air. The heat processing that occurs during canning also affects vitamin C, but sometimes the manufacturer will add extra and this will be stated on the can's printed label.

How can I best preserve vitamin C when cooking fresh vegetables?

Vegetables should be prepared immediately before they are used. Cook them in the minimum amount of boiling salted water, or, even better, steam them, for as little time as necessary. Do not leave vegetables soaking in the cooking water, and serve immediately. Prolonged cooking and keeping them hot can destroy almost all the vitamin C content. The best way to prepare potatoes is to bake them in their skins. Never add sodium bicarbonate to the water to improve the color of vegetables—this reduces the vitamin C value, too. Even cutting and slicing them does this, as does cooking in copper or iron pans. The best way to eat vegetables is raw.

I have heard that smokers and heavy drinkers should take extra vitamin C. Is this true?

It has been found that levels of vitamin C are lower in heavy smokers or drinkers whose diet is otherwise adequate. If you are a heavy smoker or drinker, it would seem a reasonable precaution to take more than the basic recommended daily allowance of vitamin C.

Vitamin C is considered to be one of the most vital vitamins. However, it is not enough just to eat the right foods—they must be properly prepared too, otherwise the vitamin content may be sharply reduced or lost altogether.

Vitamin C is probably the most controversial of all the vitamins. Great claims have been made for its healing and protective powers in connection with the common cold, aging, heart disease, and many other conditions. The official view remains skeptical, but no one denies that even in affluent societies people are more likely to be deficient in vitamin C than in any other nutrient.

Vitamin C is vital for maintenance of the body's connective tissue—the skin, fibers, membranes, and so on that literally hold it together. Collagen, a protein that is important for the formation of healthy skin, tendons, and bones, depends partly on vitamin C for its manufacture (see Protein; Tendons), and the vitamin is also needed for the release of hormones and the production of other chemical substances that play a part in human survival and resistance to infection (see Hormones).

Deficiency of vitamin C

The extreme form of vitamin C deficiency is a condition called scurvy, in which the connective tissue disintegrates so that blood vessels break down and there is bleeding into the skin and joints, and from the gums. Teeth are loosened, bruises appear, and resistance to infection is lowered.

Scurvy was one of the earliest deficiency diseases to be discovered. In 1497, the Portuguese navigator Vasco da Gama lost more than half his men through its effects, owing to the inevitable shortage of fresh fruit and vegetables on long voyages. In 1753, the British naval surgeon James Lind showed that scurvy could be prevented and cured by giving victims orange and lemon juice, although he was unaware of the reason for this.

Vitamin C was not actually identified as the curative agent until 1932. The name "ascorbic acid" (used to describe vitamin C when it is manufactured) comes from the term "antiscorbutic," meaning the ability to prevent and cure scurvy. This deficiency can be cured very quickly with high doses of vitamin C, but if the condition is neglected there could be permanent damage.

Vitamin C sources

Rose hips are the richest natural source of vitamin C available. Paprika is good, too, but neither of these sources of vitamin C is on everyone's daily menu, so other sources have to be relied on. Vegetables such as potatoes, which do feature

▲ *Fruit is rich in vitamin C, especially citrus fruits like oranges, lemons, and limes.*

People at risk from vitamin C deficiency

Older people	perhaps living alone, existing on canned and packaged foods
Young people	perhaps in college dormitories, living on junk foods
Food faddists	advocates of macro-cereal-based diets who do not understand the body's nutritional needs
Bottle-fed babies	given cow's milk formulas without vitamin supplements or orange juice

Vitamin C in the diet

FOOD	APPROXIMATE VITAMIN C CONTENT (MICROGRAMS)
4 oz. (114 g) fresh blackberries	220
4 oz. (114 g) fresh strawberries	70
4 oz. (114 g) lemon juice	60
1 fresh orange	60
4 oz. (114 g) canned orange juice	40
Half grapefruit	20
4 oz. (114 g) canned pineapple	12
4 oz. (114 g) boiled brussels sprouts	40
4 oz. (114 g) boiled cabbage	24
4 oz. (114 g) frozen peas	12
4 oz. (114 g) raw green peppers	112
4 oz. (114 g) boiled potatoes (according to season; new potatoes contain most)	4–20
1 fresh tomato	10

Daily vitamin C requirements

The requirements for different age groups is given in micrograms (1,000 micrograms = 1 milligram, or one-thousandth of a gram).

Babies under 12 months	30–35
Children 1–10 years	40–45
Adolescents 11–18 years	65–75
Adults	75–90
Expectant and lactating mothers/smokers	115

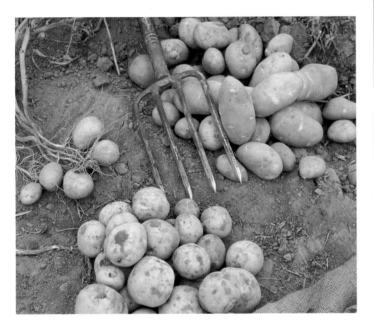

▲ *Potatoes are easy to prepare and packed with vitamin C.*

in most people's diets in the Western world, contain some vitamin C, as do brussels sprouts, cauliflower, and cabbage. Among fruits, black currants are best, followed by strawberries. Further down on the list, but available all year round, are citrus fruits (oranges, lemons, limes, and grapefruit). Rose hip syrup is obviously brimming with vitamin C, and is available from most health food stores (see Health Foods).

There is not much vitamin C in apples or pears, virtually none in milk (though it is sometimes added), and none in cereal grains, dried peas and beans, nuts, or dried fruit (the drying process rids fruit of any vitamin value). All green and root vegetables and fruit contain a certain amount, but this varies from season to season. For example, new potatoes contain three times as much vitamin C as old ones.

When extra vitamin C is needed

Some distinguished experts maintain that people need far more than the normally recommended daily allowances of vitamin C. It is generally acknowledged that the body requires additional vitamin C after a severe illness or injury, and there have been experiments showing that burns heal faster when a vitamin C solution has been applied to the skin in conjunction with injections or doses taken by mouth (see Burns).

High doses of vitamin C have also been used successfully in experiments carried out to reduce levels of cholesterol in the arteries (see Arteries and Artery Disease), and it is thought that the vitamin might offer protection against gastric bleeding in those who have to take large regular amounts of aspirin for such conditions as arthritis.

It is now known that many disease processes are ultimately mediated by what is ordinarily called oxidative stress. Highly active chemical groups called free radicals, generated by environmental processes such as toxic pollutants, radiation, and smoking, operate damagingly in many forms of pathology and can form dangerous chain reactions in tissues (see Environmental Hazards; Smoking). Vitamin C, like vitamin E, is a strong antioxidant and has the power to "mop up" free radicals. Medical research has shown that high levels of vitamin C help reduce some of the major killing diseases, especially heart attacks and strokes.

Too much vitamin C

The body excretes any surplus of vitamin C and any massive dose that is not utilized by the body is flushed away in urine, so there is no possibility of an overdose. However, people seem to be able to function normally and healthily on small amounts.

See also: **Antioxidants; Bones; Common cold; Diet; Food additives; Scurvy; Vitamins**

Vitamin D

Questions and Answers

Will sitting under a sunlamp give me enough vitamin D?

No. You will get some vitamin D, but not as much as you need. Diet is much more important, and you must make sure that yours contains sufficient vitamin D. However, some people with seasonal affective disorder (SAD) claim that using a sunlamp is an effective treatment, and it is possible that SAD is related to a deficiency in vitamin D.

I sunbathe in the yard when the weather permits. Do I need to worry about getting enough vitamin D in my diet as well?

If you lived, say, in Hong Kong, you could afford not to worry about vitamin D in your diet. There, the average diet is low in vitamin D, but signs of deficiency are rare because of the higher-than-average annual amounts of sunshine. However, people who live in temperate climates get less sunshine, so diet is important. If you try to eat a helping of canned fish or oily fish such as herring once a week at least, you should get enough vitamin D.

My son is going on a trip to southern Europe in August. For how long will he benefit from the vitamin D he converts there?

The body can store vitamin D for several months. In the northern hemisphere, the highest rates are found in the blood in September. A survey of children who had spent some weeks at the coast in summer showed that they had much higher reserves of vitamin D as compared with children who had not; these reserves were still present the following February. While sunshine is good for you, you also need to be aware of the damage that can ensue from staying out too long in the hot sun without taking precautions.

The sunshine vitamin, vitamin D, helps the body to absorb calcium and so is essential for the normal growth and development of a child's bones, and for the maintenance of healthy bones in an adult.

Vitamin D is sometimes called the sunshine vitamin because humans derive part of their essential supplies from exposure to the sun. People also obtain it from food, but there is some danger of deficiency, since it does not occur in many foods. Humans need vitamin D so that they can get enough calcium to make healthy bones. Vitamin D helps the absorption of calcium and phosphorus from the intestinal wall and maintains correct levels in the bloodstream.

There are two main types of vitamin D. When people derive it from sunshine, ultraviolet rays hit the skin and convert cholesterol in the skin into cholecalciferol, or vitamin D3 (see Cholesterol). The other main kind of vitamin D is called ergocalciferol, or D2, and is manufactured from plant materials such as yeasts.

Comparatively few foods contain vitamin D. Besides cod-liver oil, it is available most richly in herrings, kippers, canned salmon, and sardines. If a person thinks he or she is not taking a sufficient amount, supplies of vitamin D can be increased with a daily spoonful of cod-liver oil or a helping of canned fish once or twice a week. Margarine is required to have vitamin D added to it during production, and evaporated milk usually has extra, too. Butter and fresh milk have much

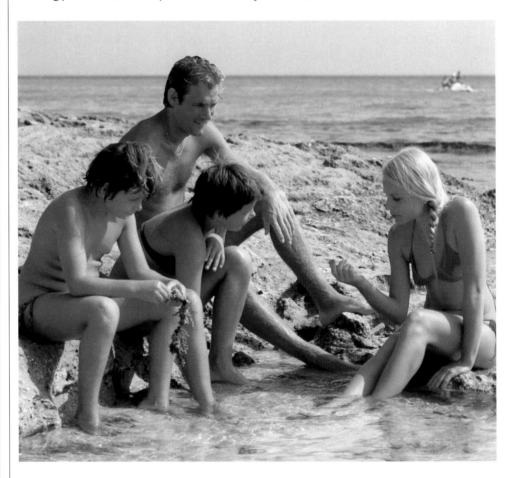

▲ *People need to be aware that the ultraviolet rays in sunlight can be both beneficial and harmful to health. Vitamin D is crucial to the body's production of vitamin D; at the same time, ultraviolet rays can cause serious long-term damage to the skin, including cancer. Exposure to the sun should always be regulated sensibly.*

Vitamin D: How much do you need?

It is not necessary to maintain the intake on a daily basis, but over a period of a week the intake should average out. The figures here are in micrograms (1,000 micrograms = 1 milligram or one-thousandth of a gram).

AGE RANGE	DAILY INTAKE
Children	10
Adults 19–50 years	5
Adults 51–69 years	10
Adults 70+ years	15
Pregnant and lactating women	10

Vitamin D content in foods

FOOD	VITAMIN D CONTENT
Glass of milk	0.16
Canned sardines in oil 4 oz. (114 g)	14.16
Hard cheese 2 oz. (50 g)	0.14
Cod-liver oil 1 tbsp. (15 ml)	60.00
1 egg	1.00
Fortified evaporated milk 4 fl. oz. (125 ml)	0.44
Fried liver 4 oz. (114 g)	0.44
Herring 4 oz. (114 g)	25.60
Kipper 4 oz. (114 g)	25.52
Margarine 2 oz. (50 g)	4.50

smaller amounts, but because of their use daily by most people, they are a good source. Eggs contain some vitamin D, as well.

Vitamin D deficiency

The main result of vitamin D deficiency is rickets in children. Rickets is a condition of defective bone growth. It causes bowlegs and knock-knees; the ribs also take on a distorted appearance and the chest and pelvis become narrowed (see Growth).

Early symptoms of rickets include restlessness, sweating, lack of muscle tone, and softening of the bones of the skull. The baby's teeth may be slow in appearing or may be soft and susceptible to decay. The bones are fragile and easily broken, and there may be muscle spasms and twitching. Extra vitamin D can reverse the effects if it is given early enough, but damage can be permanent. Rickets has now been virtually wiped out in the Western world.

An adult form of vitamin D deficiency is osteomalacia, which causes bone softening and breakage, muscular weakness, tenderness, and pain. The condition can affect older people if they live on a diet that is low in calcium and vitamin D. Osteomalacia is often associated with osteoporosis, which also increases risk of breakage.

Excessive vitamin D

Since vitamin D is stored in fat, any extra cannot be expelled easily from the body. Instead, it is stored in the liver and can lead to certain poisonous effects if the intake is too high. Early signs of excess vitamin D include appetite loss, nausea, and vomiting. Because vitamin D helps the absorption of calcium, too much vitamin D may cause unhealthily high concentrations of calcium in the blood, leading to brittle bones, hardening of the arteries, and growth failure in children.

In the West vitamin D, mainly in the form of D2, may be recommended for pregnant and breast-feeding women, and children under age five. Anyone taking a vitamin D supplement should follow the instructions and take no further D2 on top of the suggested dose.

See also: **Bones; Calcium; Diet; Osteoporosis; Rickets; Teeth and teething; Vitamins**

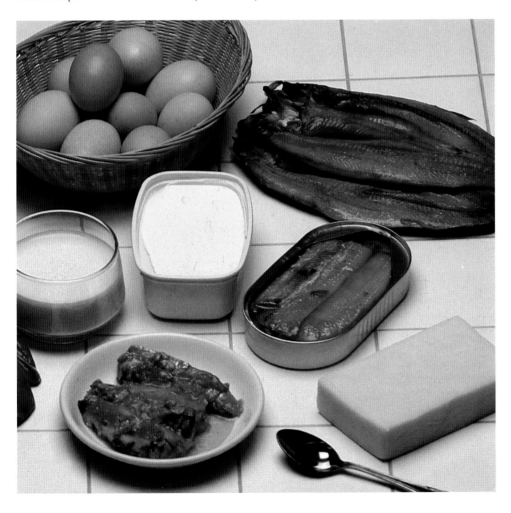

▲ *People living in temperate climates must get a proportion of the vitamin D they need in their diet. It can be found in foods such as oily fish, milk, eggs, and hard cheese.*

Vitamin E

Should I give my family muesli for breakfast? I have heard that it contains a lot of vitamin E.

It depends on the muesli. Look at the label on the packet to see if the contents include whole or rolled oats, nuts, and sesame seeds; all these contain vitamin E.

Does vitamin E improve sexual performance?

Vitamin E does have this reputation, but there has yet to be definite proof. Possibly the greatest benefit is psychological.

Could my iron pills interfere with my ability to absorb vitamin E?

Medications containing iron work against the absorption of vitamin E. Therefore, iron should be taken at a different time of day—in the morning if vitamin E is taken in any extra form in the evening. Mineral oils such as castor oil, taken as a laxative, impair absorption of vitamin E and other nutrients. Estrogen in the contraceptive pill and in hormone replacement therapy may impair absorption. Some people taking iron or estrogen have a daily teaspoon of wheat-germ oil, though this is probably not necessary.

Should I use vegetable oils in my cooking as a source of vitamin E?

In theory, yes, since these oils contain vitamin E, but a high intake of polyunsaturated vegetable oils creates an increased need for the vitamin. This is because the presence of other fats restricts the absorption of vitamin E. Polyunsaturated fats may be recommended for patients with high cholesterol levels, since the fats help reduce these levels, but more vitamin E is needed to maintain a balance.

Research into the benefits of vitamin E is still in progress, but some people claim that it has remarkable curative and rejuvenating powers. It is the antioxidant powers of vitamin E that are of particular interest.

Until the last few decades, vitamin E was not of any particular interest, largely because doctors have tended to be been mainly focused on the effects of vitamin deficiency; and vitamin E deficiency is very rare. However, a new and exciting role for this neglected vitamin has appeared.

It was believed that the fat-soluble vitamin E was unimportant. Some people have even gone so far as to say that vitamin E is of no medical relevance in humans. These views have now undergone a radical change.

History

In 1922, it was discovered that female rats required an unknown substance in their diets to sustain normal pregnancies. Without this substance, they could ovulate and conceive normally, but within about 10 days the fetus died and was absorbed. Male rats deficient in this substance were also found to have abnormalities in their testes.

The unknown substance turned out to be a new vitamin, and was given the designation "vitamin E." Fourteen years later it was chemically isolated from wheat-germ oil, and was found

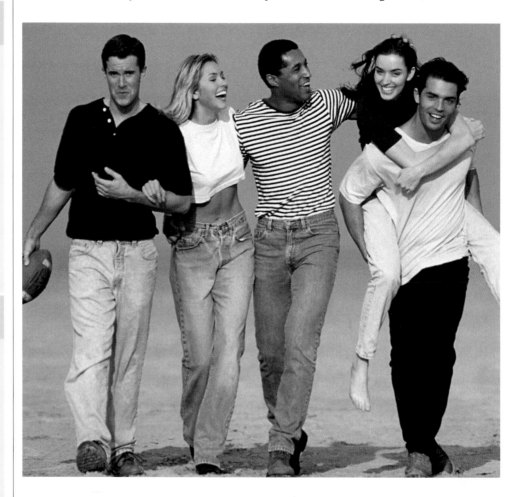

▲ *Vitamin E can help keep skin young and healthy-looking. Eating a sensible balanced diet should provide enough vitamin E, but supplements, in the form of either capsules or lotions, can also be taken.*

to be one of a range of eight very complicated but similar molecules known as tocopherols.

The news of the availability of the new vitamin was greeted with interest, and, for a time, vitamin E enjoyed a reputation as a vitamin that could be used to treat sterility. Doctors prescribed vitamin E freely as a treatment for infertility (see Infertility), although this was illogical: there was no reason to suppose that the people concerned were deficient in the vitamin.

Erroneous use

In the same way that other vitamins were used to treat deficiencies, vitamin E was used, but in the belief that it could benefit, in people who were not deficient in it, those conditions caused by its deficiency. By association, vitamin E was also used, quite mistakenly, to attempt to treat various menstrual disorders, inflammation of the vagina, and menopausal symptoms. Once it was found to be

▼ *Eggs, nuts, sunflower oil, and whole grains are good natural sources of vitamin E. If supplements are taken, they should not exceed 150 international units (IU).*

ineffective for these conditions, interest died down, and for many years the vitamin was largely forgotten.

Vitamin E deficiency

Human vitamin E deficiency is very rare because the vitamin occurs widely in many foods, and especially in vegetable oils, such as sunflower oil. Deficiency occurs only after many months on a severely restricted diet or in people who are artificially fed. A daily intake of 10 to 30 mg of the vitamin is sufficient to keep blood levels within normal limits, and this will be provided by any reasonable diet. Human milk contains enough to meet a baby's needs. In the unlikely event that deficiency does occur, however, the effects can be devastating.

Severe deficiency can cause myriad health problems: degenerative changes in the brain (see Brain Damage and Disease) and nervous system, impairment of vision (see Eyes and Eyesight), double vision, problems with walking, anemia (see Anemia), an increased rate of destruction of red blood cells, fluid retention (see Edema), and skin disorders (see Skin and Skin Diseases).

Although deficiency effects are extremely uncommon, in the last few years the reason for such devastating effects has become known.

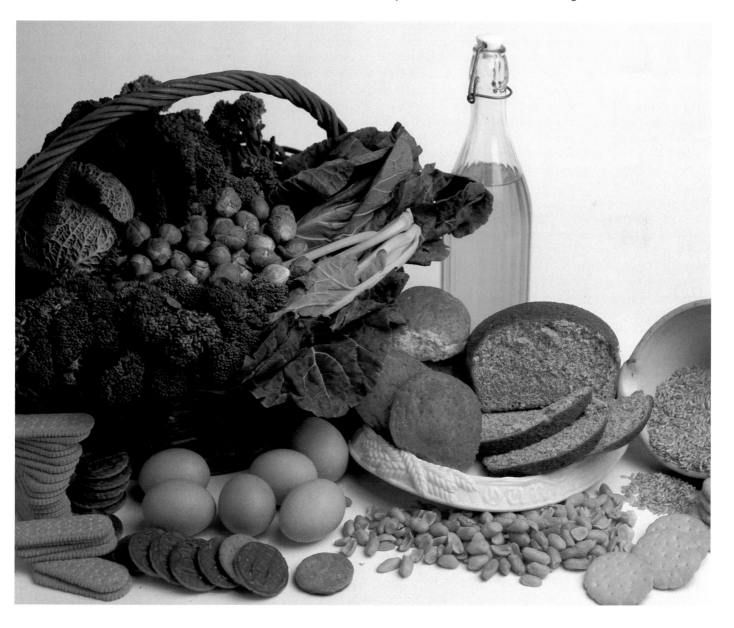

Free radicals

Chemists have known about free radicals for about 100 years, and gradually it has become apparent that they are implicated in disease. Free radicals are highly active, short-lived chemical groups that contain an atom with an unpaired outer orbital electron. The stable state is a pair of electrons, and if only one is present the atom will quickly capture an electron from a nearby atom, causing molecular damage or oxidation. When this happens the deprived atom forms a free radical. In this way a chain reaction can be set up that can quickly damage tissues. For many years, chemists have known that free radical oxidation action can be controlled, or even prevented, by a range of antioxidant substances. Antioxidants are used to prevent lubricating oils from drying up, and to protect plastics from free radical damage.

Foodstuffs have long been protected from free radical damage by antioxidants. When fat goes rancid it does so by a free radical oxidation reaction. This can be prevented by additives with antioxidant properties such as BHA (butylated hydroxyanisole), BHT (butylated hydroxytoluene), and tocopherol (vitamin E).

Natural body antioxidants

Medical interest in the possibility that free radicals were involved in disease processes was aroused when it was discovered that the body has its own natural antioxidants. One of the most effective of these is vitamin E. This vitamin is especially important because it is fat-soluble and much of the most significant free radical damage in the body is damage to the membranes of cells and to low-density lipoproteins. Vitamin C is also a powerful antioxidant, but it is soluble in water, not in fat. Therefore, it is distributed to all parts of the body. Vitamins C and E are highly efficient at mopping up free radicals, and work together to do this (see Vitamin C).

The tocopherols

Among the richest natural sources of the tocopherols are seed germ oils, alfalfa, and lettuce. They are widely distributed in plant materials. Tocopherols are almost insoluble in water but dissolve in oils, fats, alcohol, acetone, ether, and other fat solvents. Unlike vitamin C they are stable to heat and alkalis in the absence of oxygen, and are unaffected by acids at temperatures up to 212°F (100°C). Because vitamin E consists of so many slightly different tocopherols, worldwide standardization is difficult and a little arbitrary. The

Good sources of vitamin E

Figures are given as the number of micrograms in 100 grams (3.527 ounces)

Bran	2,000
Almonds, shelled	2,000
Butter	2,000
Cornflakes	400
Potato chips	6,100
Eggs	1,600
Hazelnuts, shelled	2,100
Peanuts, fresh or roasted	8,100
Muesli	3,200
Sunflower oil	1,800
Whole wheat bread	200

Vitamin E—How much do you need?

United States recommended daily allowances are as follows.

AGE RANGE	mg
Babies up to 6 months	3–4
Children 6 months to 8 years	6–7
Children 9–13 years	11
Adolescents 14+ and adults	15
Lactating women	19

international unit of vitamin E is taken to be equal to 1 mg of alpha-tocopherol acetate. For practical purposes of dosage, however, 1.5 international units (IU) is considered to be equivalent to 1 mg.

Antioxidant properties

All the tocopherols have antioxidant properties and this appears to be the basis for all the biological effects of the vitamin. The effects of vitamin E deficiency are, it seems, the effects of inadequate antioxidant protection. Vitamin E is involved in many body processes, and, in conjunction with vitamin C, operates as a natural antioxidant, helping to protect important cell structures, especially cell membranes, from the damaging effects of free radicals. In animals, vitamin E supplements can protect against the effects of various drugs, chemicals, and metals that can promote free radical formation. In carrying out its function as an antioxidant in the body, vitamin E is, itself, converted to a radical. It is, however, soon regenerated to the active vitamin by a biochemical process that probably involves both vitamin C and another natural body antioxidant, glutathione.

Dangers of overdosage

Publicity about the antioxidant value of vitamins E and C has led many people to take these vitamins on a regular daily basis, sometimes as part of an organized therapy. Like vitamin C, vitamin E is generally regarded as a fairly innocuous substance and few if any warnings are heard of the dangers of overdosage (see Overdoses). For adults, this is probably reasonable, but there are limits to the amounts that can be safely taken and recommended dosages should not be exceeded.

Vitamin E and babies

There is, however, a special caveat in the case of babies. Although free radicals are generally destructive, the body also uses them for beneficial purposes. They are, for instance, the mechanism by which phagocyte cells destroy bacteria (see Bacteria). This action is unlikely to be interfered with in adults, but it is known that dangers have arisen from overdosage of vitamin E in premature babies (see Premature Babies). Large doses of vitamin E have been shown to interfere sufficiently with the action of the cells of the immune system to cause a dangerous form of intestinal infection (see Digestive System). For this reason, doses of supplementary vitamin E should never be given to babies except under strict medical supervision.

See also: Antioxidants; Diet; Nervous system; Vitamins

Vitamin K

By helping the blood to clot, vitamin K performs a vital function in the body. A balanced diet provides some of the vitamin K required by the body, and deficiencies are rare and usually easily treated.

Vitamin K consists of vitamin K1, a yellow oil found in a variety of vegetables; and vitamin K2, a yellow waxy substance produced by bacteria. Although vitamin K1 is abundant in leafy vegetables such as spinach and green cabbage, a normal diet will provide only a proportion of the daily requirement. The remainder of vitamin K2 is obtained from bacteria that live in the intestines, and this ensures that there is always a steady supply. In healthy people a deficiency resulting from an inadequate diet is rare.

Vitamin K deficiency

Vitamin K is used by the liver to produce three of the blood components known as the clotting factors (see Liver and Liver Diseases). A deficiency results in a decreased production of these three factors. The most important clotting factor is prothrombin. When an injury occurs, the ability of the blood to coagulate will be impaired. Small cuts will bleed vigorously, and large bruises will form under the skin in response to even minor injuries. In severe cases of vitamin K deficiency, serious and even fatal hemorrhaging may occur (see Hemorrhage). Because vitamins K1 and K2 are fat-soluble

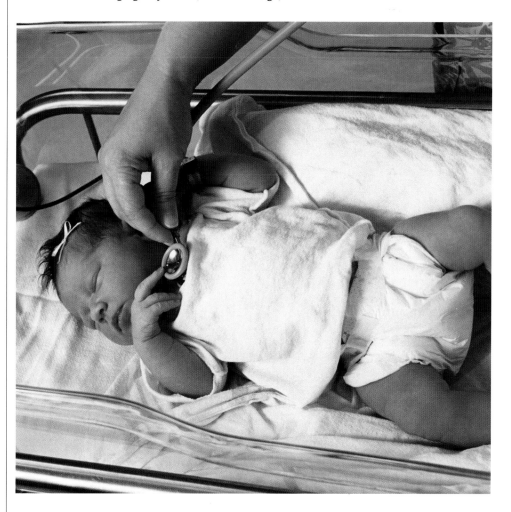

▲ *Babies may be given vitamin K at birth because they have no intestinal bacteria to produce it and the supply from the mother's bloodstream is quickly depleted.*

Vitamin K—How much do you need?

The figures below are only rough estimates. Daily requirement cannot be calculated accurately, because so much of Vitamin K intake is supplied by intestinal bacteria. The figures given below are in micrograms (1,000 micrograms = 1 milligram, or one-thousandth of a gram).

AGE GROUP	DAILY REQUIREMENT
Babies up to 1 year	5–10
Children under ten years	15–30
Adolescent men (11–18 years)	45–65
Adolescent women (11–18 years)	45–55
Adult men (19+)	70–80
Adult women (19+)	60–65

Vitamin K content of food

Figures given are micrograms per 100 gm (3.53 oz) of food.

Lean meat	100–200
Cows' liver	100–200
Pigs' liver	400–800
Eggs (each)	20
Cows' milk	2
Human breast milk	20
Potatoes	80
Spinach	4,200
Green cabbage	3,200
Carrots	100
Peas	100–300
Tomatoes	400

(they are dissolved and stored in fat), a deficiency may occur in diseases that cause decreased digestion and absorption of fats and oils (see Fats). These include an obstruction of the bile duct and celiac disease (see Celiac Disease). This deficiency can easily be treated with vitamin K injections or with pills containing synthetic vitamin K. Some liver diseases, such as cirrhosis of the liver and hepatitis (see Cirrhosis; Hepatitis), interfere with the utilization of vitamin K, and vitamin supplements in large doses may then be required. A deficiency is sometimes difficult to treat and can be dangerous in patients with liver failure, who may develop uncontrollable internal bleeding.

Finally, vitamin K deficiency is often found in the newborn, and may cause serious damage both from blood loss and from bleeding into the brain and other vital organs. Intestinal bacteria are not present at birth; milk contains very little vitamin K; and the supply from the mother's bloodstream does not last long. To make up this deficiency, some newborn babies are given a small shot of vitamin K.

Excess vitamin K

Vitamin K is nontoxic (that is, not poisonous) if taken in excessive amounts because the liver controls the rate of production of the clotting factors. Some patients have an increased tendency to thrombosis, (formation of blood clots; see Thrombosis). These blood clots obstruct the healthy blood vessels in which they are first formed, and may also be carried around the body in the bloodstream to obstruct blood vessels elsewhere. The limbs, lungs, brain, and heart may suffer serious damage. Thrombosis is not caused by excess vitamin K, but in such patients, further blood clot formation can be prevented by taking drugs such as warfarin that stop the liver from using vitamin K to produce clotting factors.

See also: **Bile; Diet; Vitamins**

▼ *These foods supply some of the daily requirement of vitamin K, which is required to help blood to clot. The body also manufactures the vitamin to ensure a good supply.*

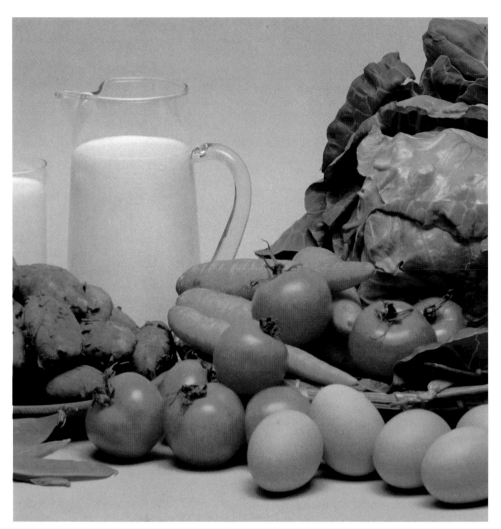

Vitamins

Questions and Answers

What are vitamins and how important are they?

Vitamins are organic substances present in minute amounts in food. They help make our bodies work. Because they cannot be made in the body, vitamins must be obtained from the diet or from sunshine. We require only small amounts, but they are nevertheless essential to normal metabolism, and a serious deficiency will lead to disease.

I have very low energy levels. Might I have a vitamin deficiency?

It is most unlikely that a person on a normal diet would suffer a vitamin deficiency. Although it is possible that you are depressed, vitamins are unlikely to help. The only time extra vitamins should be taken is when you are on an abnormal or restricted diet.

My hair has started to fall out, and I now have bald patches. Could this be a vitamin problem?

It is unlikely. Hair has cycles of growth and rest, and it is normal to notice more hair loss at some times than others. What is more, any number of conditions or factors can be responsible for hair loss and baldness—from alopecia to overperming. It would be a good idea to seek medical advice.

Can taking too many vitamins be harmful?

Taking too much vitamin A and D can be harmful. Too much vitamin A can result in fragile bones, liver and spleen enlargement, and loss of appetite. Overdoses of vitamin D can cause vomiting, headache, weight loss, and calcium deposits in the kidneys and arteries. Always follow your doctor's dosage recommendations when taking vitamin supplements.

Everyone knows that vitamins are important and that a deficiency can cause illness. However, there is more to the vitamin story than that, and there have been some interesting and important developments in recent years.

Vitamins are chemical compounds necessary for normal body function. Nearly everything that happens in the body is mediated by chemical activators called enzymes, and vitamins are essential components in many of the enzyme systems of the body. Vitamins operate within the cells, assisting in the synthesis of tissue-building material, hormones, and chemical regulators; they participate in energy production; and they assist in the breakdown of waste products and toxic substances. The B group of vitamins, for instance, function as coenzymes, substances without which the vital enzyme-accelerated chemical processes of the body cannot occur or do so abnormally.

In general, people get all the vitamins they need from a normal, well-balanced diet. The quantities needed for health are very small. With the exception of vitamins C and E,

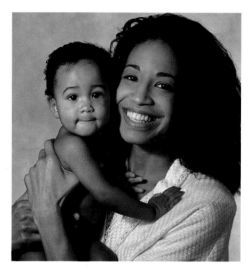

▲ *Mothers and babies, in particular, benefit from a balanced, vitamin-rich diet.*

vitamins taken in excess of the minimum requirement are simply wasted. In the case of vitamins A and D, excessive intake can actually be dangerous and even fatal.

Vitamin deficiency is uncommon in well-nourished populations, but can occur in people on fad diets or those practicing extreme forms of vegetarianism; in people with malabsorption disorders; in alcoholics who get enough calories from alcohol and who feel no need to eat; and in people taking certain drugs, such as hydralazine, penicillamine, and estrogens.

Vitamins are conventionally divided into the fat-soluble group A, D, E, and K; and the water-soluble group, vitamin C (ascorbic acid) and the B vitamins. Because of their metabolic function, they are found in highest concentration in the most metabolically active parts of animal and plant tissues, the liver, and seed germs.

Recent developments

A recent development in the field is the recognition that vitamins C and E have properties that are distinct from their previously known functions. Both vitamins are powerful antidioxidants, and there is increasing evidence that large daily doses have substantial health benefits.

The new knowledge is that the immediate cause of much tissue damage in disease and environmental injury is the action of destructive chemical groups known as oxygen free radicals. Research has shown that doses of the order of 1,000 milligrams of C and 400 milligrams of E can have the effect of mopping up free radicals and preventing them from causing molecular damage.

In particular, it is now becoming widely accepted that the mechanisms of arterial damage leading to the deposition of cholesterol and other material in the lining of arteries involves free radical action. Research projects are increasingly supporting the probability that the resulting disease, atherosclerosis, which leads to heart attacks and strokes, can be countered by regular large supplements of antioxidant vitamins.

Atherosclerosis is the cause of more premature deaths and severe morbidity in developed countries than all other major diseases put together.

See also: Alcoholism; Cholesterol; Diet; Enzymes; Hormones; Vegetarianism

Vitiligo

Questions and Answers

I have white spots developing on my hands. Could this be vitiligo?

Yes, possibly. Vitiligo usually starts as small white spots on skin exposed to the sun, like the backs of the hands. If vitiligo is going to develop, the spots enlarge and run into each other, perhaps over a few months. Vitiligo is not serious, but it would be wise to consult your doctor about it.

Is vitiligo inherited?

Yes. Though there is no definite pattern of inheritance, about 30 percent of sufferers have a family history of the condition.

Vitiligo appeared on my face and hands some years ago, and now I have been told my thyroid is failing. Is there a connection?

Yes. Vitiligo seems to be associated with all the autoimmune diseases of hormone glands. In an autoimmune disease, the body's immune system turns against its own tissue. Vitiligo can be associated with failure of the thyroid and of the adrenal glands, and it can also be associated with pernicious anemia. More than one of these diseases can occur in the same patient, and the fact that all these problems tend to occur together has led to the suggestion that vitiligo, too, is an autoimmune disease. Doctors believe this to be the case, but there is no proof.

Does vitiligo ever get better?

A small number of people regain their skin color, but the condition is unlikely to improve much once the pigment has been lost. However, the disease is no more than a cosmetic embarrassment, and the only problem is an increased risk of sunburn. Makeup can conceal any unsightly patches.

Vitiligo causes pale patches, due to loss of melanin, to appear on the skin, usually on the face and hands. Though these can be unsightly and distressing, vitiligo is not a serious disease.

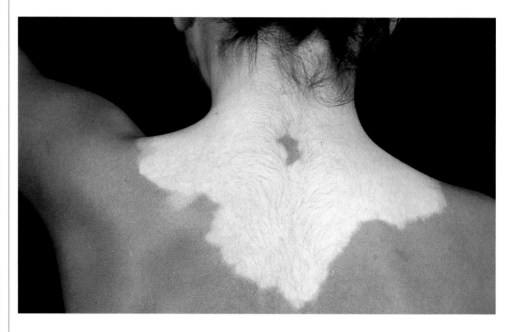

▲ *Although not a serious threat to health, the patchy loss of pigment that is the characteristic symptom of vitiligo can cause a considerable amount of distress.*

Vitiligo is a condition in which areas of skin lose their pigment and show up as very pale patches. The disease does not seriously affect health, but it can cause a cosmetic problem to a sufferer. Vitiligo is not uncommon: it may occur in as many as 1 percent of the world's population. Although many people are affected, the extent of the problem is often very slight. It seems that women are more likely than men to seek advice, mainly for cosmetic reasons, but in fact the overall incidence may actually be the same in both sexes.

Causes and symptoms

Although vitiligo can be occupationally acquired, most doctors favor the theory that vitiligo is mainly an autoimmune disease: that is, one in which the body's own immune system has attacked another part of the body. Since vitiligo is an autoimmune disorder, it is likely that antibodies are produced to cells that produce melanin (see Melanin).

The disease has one effect, the loss of pigmentation on the skin. Usually this is found in areas that are exposed to sun, such as the backs of the hands, although eventually it may become more widespread. The depigmented areas of skin start as small areas, which then run together to produce enlarging areas of pale skin. The areas around the depigmented skin may be more heavily pigmented than usual. About half of the sufferers start losing pigment before they reach age 20. The pale areas may develop quite quickly over the course of a few months, and then remain unchanged for years. Hair growing in pale areas may also gradually lose its color.

Treatment

There is no cure. Drugs called psoralens have been tried, combined with phototherapy, but although there may be some improvement, there is also a risk of toxicity.

See also: **Hormones; Immune system; Skin and skin diseases; Sunburn**

Vocal cords

The vocal cords are two strong bands of tissue inside the larynx that vibrate as air exhaled from the lungs passes between them, producing the sound that is a basis for speech.

Questions and Answers

Why do boys' voices change so dramatically during puberty?

Because of the sudden growth of the larynx. This is triggered by the production of male hormones such as testosterone. The voice breaks, dropping in pitch as the larynx grows and the vocal cords lengthen. The tone of the voice is probably inherited.

I have been told that I must have a laryngectomy. What is it, and will I be able to speak afterward?

A laryngectomy is the removal of the larynx and the vocal cords, usually as a result of cancer. A small round hole is made in the neck and windpipe so that the patient can breathe. The hole is known as a tracheostomy, and the larynx and the surrounding malignant tissue are removed. After the removal of the vocal cords, any voice produced must be artificial; this can be achieved in a number of ways. Esophageal speech can be learned by swallowing air into the stomach and belching in a controlled manner. Or artificial vocal cords can be used in the form of a small vibrator that is placed on the neck at the site of the removed Adam's apple. When the patient exhales and mouths the words, artificial vibration of the air coming through the throat produces a functional if rather monotonous metallic voice. Such devices have been improved in recent years. With practice, they can be used to produce almost natural voice tones.

I lost my voice and now have a rasping cough. What should I do?

If you smoke, quit; it worsens the condition. Try not to speak for a few days. Steam inhalations may help, but if the condition does not improve in two weeks, see the doctor.

POSITION AND STRUCTURE OF THE VOCAL CORDS

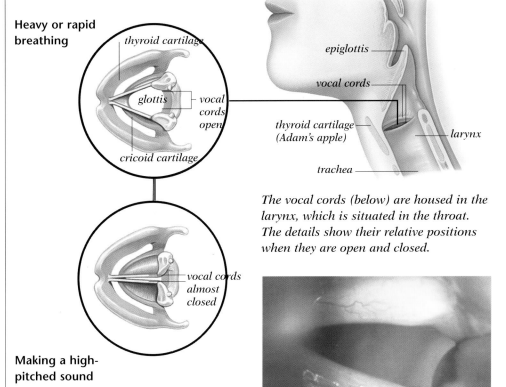

Heavy or rapid breathing

thyroid cartilage

glottis

vocal cords open

cricoid cartilage

epiglottis

vocal cords

thyroid cartilage (Adam's apple)

larynx

trachea

vocal cords almost closed

Making a high-pitched sound

The vocal cords (below) are housed in the larynx, which is situated in the throat. The details show their relative positions when they are open and closed.

The vocal cords are similar to the reed in a wind instrument such as a bassoon. When a musician blows air between the reeds, the thin wood strips vibrates, producing the basic sound that is modified by the pipe length and holes of the instrument. Similarly, the vocal cords vibrate when someone vocalizes, and the sounds produced are modified by the throat, nose, and mouth.

The vocal cords are in the larynx. They consist of two delicate ligaments, shaped like lips, which open and close as air passes through them. One end is attached to a pair of movable cartilages called the arytenoids; the other is anchored to the thyroid cartilage, which is part of the Adam's apple. The arytenoid cartilages alter position so that the space between the cords (the rima) varies in shape from a narrow V during speech to a closed slit during swallowing.

The vibration of the vocal cords during speech occurs when the rima narrows and air from the lungs is expelled between the cords and through the larynx. The loudness of the voice is controlled by the force with which air is expelled, and the pitch by the length and tension of the cords. The depth and timbre of the voice are due to the shape and size of the throat, nose, and mouth. Men usually have a large larynx, longer vocal cords, and deeper voices than women.

Disorders of the vocal cords cause hoarseness due to inflammation of the larynx. It can occur as a result of cheering at a football game or a viral infection such as a cold. Laryngeal tumors may cause laryngitis: they are usually benign polyps, cysts, or growths known as singers' nodes because of constant rubbing of the vocal cords, and have to be surgically removed.

See also: Larynx and laryngitis; Speech

Vomiting

Questions and Answers

What is the best first aid treatment for vomiting?

Avoid solid foods that could make you vomit more. Drink plenty of bland fluids—water or sips of soda—and avoid alcohol. If you cannot keep fluids down, suck ice cubes. A teaspoonful of baking soda diluted in a teacup of water or milk can help. As you feel better, eat dry bread, soups, and custards. Return to your normal diet over three or four days.

I have heard people say that they had almost vomited up their insides. Can this really happen?

No. This just describes a severe bout. If the vomiting is caused by food poisoning or severe gastroenteritis it can be extremely unpleasant and distressing. No matter how violently or persistently you vomit, there is no possibility at all that you will bring up your internal organs.

Is it necessary always to see your doctor about vomiting?

No. Vomiting usually lasts for only a day or two and has an obvious cause. If you get regular bouts of vomiting, or have abdominal pain, or if you have recently had a blow on the head, or if there is a possibility that you may be pregnant, you should see your doctor. If the vomit contains blood, go to your doctor immediately.

I have had repeated vomiting bouts, and I am to go and have tests. What is involved?

After initial examination by your doctor, you may be sent for an endoscopic examination of your stomach. You may see a gastroenterologist, who may look in your stomach with an endoscope. The tests are simple and should cause you no pain.

Vomiting may be accompanied by nausea, dizziness, and faintness—it is an exhausting and unpleasant experience, but it is a mechanism of survival that warns us of danger.

Vomiting is the forceful ejection of the contents of the stomach through the mouth, and it is an unpleasant and often exhausting experience. It can be caused by many conditions and is usually triggered by the middle ear, gastrointestinal tract, or brain. The condition may be brought on by motion sickness, food poisoning, or unpleasant odors or sights. Sometimes it is a symptom of a more serious complaint, such as a heart attack or cancer.

The actual mechanism causing the ejection of food is straightforward. At the onset of vomiting, the pylorus (a muscular valve through which food normally passes from the stomach into the intestines) closes (see Digestive System). The waves of stomach contractions that normally push food downward into the intestines reverse, pressure inside the stomach builds up, the larynx (windpipe) closes, and the muscles of the abdominal wall contract suddenly, forcing the contents of the stomach to burst up through the esophagus and out of the mouth. Three main areas of the body, when stimulated, can bring about vomiting; although the mechanism is the same in each case, the causes are different.

Stomach irritation

Irritation of the stomach lining is the most common cause of vomiting. This can be brought on by a surprising variety of conditions, including gastritis, gastroenteritis (see Gastroenteritis), peritonitis (see Peritoneum), appendicitis (see Appendicitis), and ulcers (see Ulcers); tonsillitis can also cause vomiting in young children (see Tonsils). These types of complaint are associated with viral infections and inflammation, and should be treated as soon as possible by a doctor. The most common cause of stomach irritation is eating or drinking to excess, or eating contaminated or impure food (see Food Poisoning). The body protects itself against potential harm by expelling dangerous substances. A bout of vomiting is usually short-lived, lasting only a day or two, and is

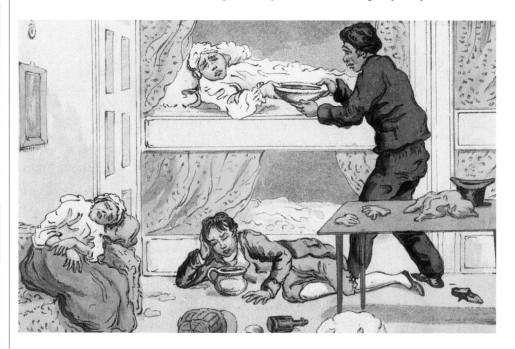

▲ *Seasickness is a common complaint. This detail from a 19th-century caricature shows some wretched passengers on a transport ship and accurately illustrates the misery of motion sickness.*

MECHANISM OF VOMITING

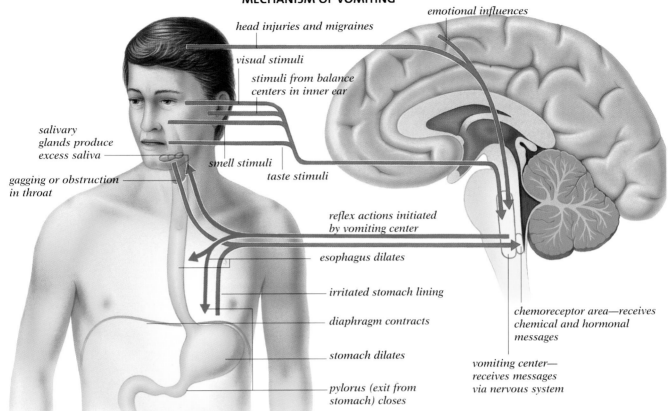

head injuries and migraines

emotional influences

visual stimuli

stimuli from balance
centers in inner ear

salivary
glands produce
excess saliva

smell stimuli

taste stimuli

gagging or obstruction
in throat

reflex actions initiated
by vomiting center

esophagus dilates

irritated stomach lining

diaphragm contracts

stomach dilates

pylorus (exit from
stomach) closes

chemoreceptor area—receives
chemical and hormonal
messages

vomiting center—
receives messages
via nervous system

rarely a serious condition. Putting fingers down the back of the throat will also cause vomiting, and use is made of this reflex action in trying to make people eject certain poisonous substances. The function of the reflex is to protect the body from swallowing anything that is unsuitable. This method of induced vomiting is also used by people suffering from bulimia, in which huge quantities of food are eaten and vomiting is induced shortly afterward. This is used as a form of weight control.

The ears and motion sickness

Motion sickness is another common cause of vomiting (see Motion Sickness), resulting from contrasting information that reaches the brain from the various organs of balance: the semicircular canals in the ear. If what is seen conflicts with information received from these canals, and the brain is not able to interpret the two, it triggers impulses to the vomiting center in the brain and results in nausea and vomiting. As well as travelers, it can also afflict sufferers of Ménière's disease (see Ménière's Disease), in which the organs of hearing and balance are affected.

A blow to the head, even a light blow, can cause vomiting, and indicates serious bleeding inside the skull. The desire to vomit usually occurs sometime after the blow, even as long as two days later. It is an indication that a damaged blood vessel has allowed pressure to accumulate on the brain and around the vomiting center. This must be treated quickly, since potentially fatal brain compression may be occurring.

Vomiting also frequently occurs in pregnancy. This is called morning sickness, a form of vomiting that is not fully understood but is believed to be related to the changing level of hormones in the blood during early pregnancy (see Hormones; Pregnancy). In a few

▲ *Vomiting is a reflex action. Nerve impulses from around the body carry messages—of danger, irritation, or confusion— to the vomiting center in the brain stem. Toxic agents or hormonal changes act upon the chemoreceptor area nearby, thus also stimulating the vomiting center. At the same time, impulses passing to the cortex produce feelings of nausea. When the vomiting threshold is passed, the vomiting center initiates a number of physical changes that result in the ejection of the stomach's contents through the mouth.*

women it is persistent and severe and may necessitate a stay in the hospital (see Prenatal Care).

Repeated vomiting

Repeated bouts of vomiting are a symptom of a serious disorder and should be brought to doctor's attention immediately. The content of the vomit is also important. It will usually consist of the last meal eaten or may be almost entirely yellow-green, bitter bile. If there is any sign of blood, the implications are serious and medical advice should be sought. The blood may resemble coffee grounds, since it will have broken down in the stomach before the vomiting started.

Treatment

When vomiting persists, or is accompanied by fever and general malaise, a doctor must be consulted and the cause treated. When someone has been vomiting, solid foods should be avoided; diluted milk and plenty of water are best until the person can return to a normal diet.

See also: Anorexia and bulimia;
Diet; Nausea

Von Willebrand's disease

Von Willebrand's disease is a condition that interferes with the normal clotting of the blood. Although it is less well-known than hemophilia, it is actually a more common cause of abnormal bleeding.

Questions and Answers

My son has been diagnosed as suffering from von Willebrand's disease and the doctor says he inherited it from me and my husband. My husband and I are normal, so how can this be?

Von Willebrand's disease can be inherited in various ways. If both you and your husband are normal and passed on the disease to your son, it must be the recessive type, sometimes called type 3 von Willebrand's disease. In a recessive disorder, both parents must be carriers of the gene mutation so that the child receives two copies and will suffer from the disease. You and your husband will each have one normal and one mutated gene for the von Willebrand factor. The normal gene prevents you from having the disease.

I have mild von Willebrand's disease and have been told that pregnancy can make it worse. Should I avoid pregnancy?

Von Willebrand's disease is caused by a deficiency in the von Willebrand factor and levels of this factor actually rise during pregnancy in all women. In spite of this, women with severe von Willebrand's disease are at risk of postpartum hemorrhage, mainly as a result of the factor VIII deficiency that accompanies low levels of von Willebrand factor. Concentrates of factor VIII used for treatment also contain von Willebrand factor. Discuss this with your doctor and be clear about the level of risk before you decide on pregnancy.

I have von Willebrand's disease. Should I avoid taking aspirin?

Yes. Aspirin interferes with blood platelet adhesiveness. Since deficiency of the von Willebrand factor causes bleeding by a similar action, it should be avoided.

There are several types of von Willebrand's disease that interfere with blood clotting, but to different degrees. Von Willebrand's disease is the most common inherited bleeding disorder; about 30,000 people in the United States suffer from the condition.

Causes
The von Willebrand factor (vWF) is a protein necessary for binding together blood platelets. Unless this happens blood clotting cannot proceed normally, so there is an abnormal prolongation of the bleeding time. The gene for the von Willebrand factor is on the short arm of chromosome 12 and many

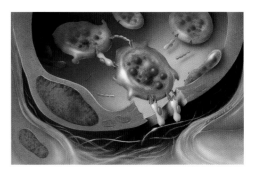

▲ *In von Willebrand's disease, a factor needed for clot formation is present at low levels or is missing from the blood.*

different mutations of this gene have been found. The vWF also acts as a carrier protein for factor VIII, the factor deficient in hemophilia, so low blood levels of factor VIII may occur in von Willebrand's disease. Some forms of the disease have dominant inheritance; others are recessive.

Symptoms
The symptoms of von Willebrand's disease are usually less severe than those of hemophilia. Spontaneous bleeding into joints and muscles, which occurs in hemophilia, is unusual, and if it does happen it is usually the result of low levels of factor VIII. Dangerous degrees of bleeding and death from hemorrhage are very rare. The most common symptoms are spontaneous nose-bleeds, prolonged bleeding after minor cuts or other trauma or surgical operations, bleeding into the skin and mucous membranes, excessively heavy menstrual periods, and severe and prolonged bleeding after childbirth. In the most common forms of the disease, the levels of vWF rise to normal after adolescence, often with disappearance of the symptoms.

Diagnosis
If von Willebrand's disease is suspected, measurements of the level of vWF in the blood and in platelets can be carried out. Diagnosis is also helped by knowing the genetic history, tests of platelet function, and blood levels of factor VIII.

Treatment
Treatment depends on the severity of the disease. In most cases it is sufficient to give von Willebrand factor and factor VIII to cover episodes of surgery or to treat excessive bleeding. It may be possible to avoid giving these blood products by the use of synthetic vasopressin (DDAVP), which causes a rise in factor VIII. This can be taken by nasal spray. If necessary, injections of highly purified vWF will usually correct the bleeding time for up to 12 hours. This has the additional bonus that, because vWF acts as a carrier protein for factor VIII, levels of factor VIII also rise and continue to be maintained for up to 72 hours after a single dose of vWF.

Mild cases may respond to another measure: the use of drugs such as tranexamic acid that block the breaking down of the protein fibrin which, with clumped platelets, is an important ingredient in blood clots. The use of local clotting agents such as topical thrombin, collagen fleece, or fibrin glue may be also useful. Intramuscular injections are avoided.

See also: **Hemophilia; Heredity**

Vulva

The word "vulva" describes the sexually sensitive outer region of the female reproductive system. This area is susceptible to a variety of infections that are collectively known as vulvitis.

Most prominent among the parts of the vulva are the two pairs of lips or labia. The outer and larger lips—labia majora—consist of thick folds of skin that cover and protect most of the other parts. They become thinner at the base and merge with the perineum (the skin over the area between the vulva and the anus). At the top the outer lips merge with the skin and hair on the pad of fatty tissue that covers the pubic bone, the mons pubis or mons veneris, which is often referred to as the "mound of Venus."

Within the labia majora are the labia minora or lesser lips. They join at the top to form a protective hood over the sensitive clitoris, dividing into folds that surround it. They also protect the opening to the urethra. The area between the labia minora is largely taken up by a space called the vestibule. Before a woman is sexually active, the space is mostly covered by the hymen. This varies in shape, size, and toughness, and although it is usually either torn or stretched during the first sexual intercourse, it may either be strong enough to make intercourse difficult or have been previously ruptured by strenuous exercise, masturbation, or tampons. The tags of skin that many women have around the vestibule are the remains of the hymen, and are called

STRUCTURE OF THE VULVA

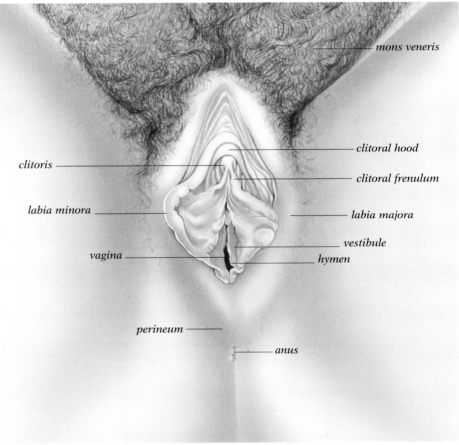

▲ *Situated at the entrance to the vagina, the vulva consists mainly of outer and inner lips called the labia. These folds of skin cover and protect the sensitive interior, including the main organ of sexual excitement—the clitoris.*

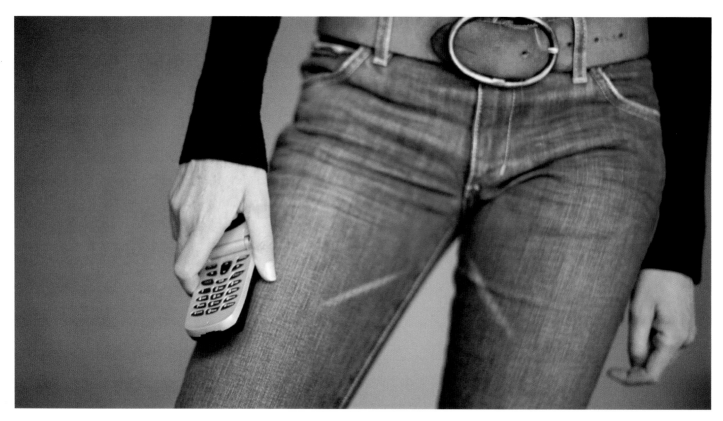

the carunculae myrtiformes. At the back the labia minora join to form the fourchette, which is often ruptured during the first childbirth (see Birth).

The clitoris and glands

The clitoris is actually similar in structure to the penis, even to the extent of having a hood of labia, the equivalent of the foreskin, and a small connecting band of tissue called the frenulum. It is primarily an organ of sexual excitement. It is extremely sensitive, and when stimulated its spongy tissue fills with blood and becomes erect. Friction on the erect clitoris—either by movement of the penis during intercourse or by some other means—will usually lead to orgasm (see Orgasm). Other parts of the vulva also respond to sexual stimulation—the labia contain erectile tissue and often become enlarged during lovemaking; and the Bartholin's glands become active. Two pairs of glands are associated with the vulva. The first are Skene's glands, which lie just below the clitoris and secrete an alkaline fluid that reduces the natural acidity of the vagina. The other, larger pair lie in the bottom of the vestibule. These are Bartholin's glands and they secrete clear mucus when a woman is sexually aroused so that the entrance to the vagina becomes lubricated and can more easily accept the penis. These glands are normally about the size of a pea and are not prominent. They are prone, however, to venereal and other infections, becoming swollen, red, and tender. This condition, called Bartholinitis, requires treatment with antibiotics. In some cases, an abscess forms in one of the glands—a Bartholin's abscess—and may need to be incised to release the pus (see Abscess; Sexually Transmitted Diseases).

Vulvitis

Vulvitis is an inflammation of the vulva or of a part of it, the labia being the structures most often involved. Although vulvitis is mostly

▲ Wearing tight-fitting jeans occasionally is fine, but if they are worn every day they can trigger vulvitis.

due to an infection, such as a yeast infection (monilia) or trichomoniasis, it can also result from the friction of tight underwear or jeans, excessive rubbing or scratching, damage from stale urine or sweat, the chemical effects of vaginal deodorants, or allergy to some material or cosmetic preparation with which it comes in contact.

Vulvitis is a likely complication of diabetes and obesity; senile vulvitis develops among the elderly as a result of decreased hormone levels (see Hormones). Currently on the increase is the form known as genital herpes, caused by infection from the herpes simplex virus (see Herpes).

Symptoms and treatment

Irrespective of cause, the symptoms of vulvitis are basically the same. The skin becomes red, sore, and itchy, and there may be some swelling. If there is a great deal of irritation, known as pruritus vulvae, scratching may make the problem worse, causing the labia to become more sore and inflamed.

In herpes, small blisters develop; these burst, leaving sore, tender ulcers that allow bacteria to penetrate the skin and cause further infection.

Treatment of vulvitis depends on the cause. It is usually necessary to consult a doctor or go to a genitourinary clinic for diagnosis and appropriate treatment. The symptoms can be relieved by wearing loose underwear or none at all, and scrupulously avoiding scratching. Also, fragranced talcum powder should be avoided, since this can exacerbate the condition.

See also: **Hygiene; Warts**

Warts

Warts are unsightly but harmless growths that can make youth a time of embarrassment. They will disappear through medical treatment or, sometimes, on their own.

Warts are a very common, usually harmless, skin affliction that affect mainly children, and to a lesser extent adults and teenagers. They consist of small rounded growths that appear on the skin and can occur virtually anywhere on the skin surface, although they are most common on the hands, knees, face, and genitals. Rarely any cause for concern, warts are usually painless and can disappear within a few months or years. However, facial and genital warts may cause some embarrassment or discomfort. They should be treated, since they can persist for years.

A type of wart that appears on the sole of the foot, commonly but wrongly known as a verruca, is often painful and also requires treatment (see Verruca).

Causes and transmission

Warts are caused by a virus called papillomavirus, which can infiltrate and multiply within the outermost layer of the skin cells. When the virus infects the skin, it causes the skin cells to

Questions and Answers

Why are warts more common among young people?

Warts are caused by a virus, to which it is possible to develop immunity so that reinfection is less likely. The strength of acquired immunity is not as great for warts as for other common childhood viral infections, such as measles or chicken pox, but because of immunity many people who had warts during childhood have a built-in defense against the infection as adults.

What is the difference between warts and verrucas?

The word "verruca" is the correct medical term for a wart, regardless of its appearance, location, or shape. "Verruca" is an abbreviation of the medical term "verruca plantaris" which means "wart on the sole." These warts are different from warts elsewhere on the body because they are pressed into the foot and usually surrounded or partly covered by a thick layer of skin.

Can warts be dangerous and do they lead to further complications?

Most warts are harmless, but warts in the genital area can obstruct the vagina, anus, or penile orifice, and wartlike growths in the throat may cause obstruction to breathing. Very rarely a wart may develop from a benign growth into a malignant or cancerous one which requires urgent surgical removal.

Is it true that childhood warts should not be treated?

Warts on the hands or knees are best left alone, since they may disappear within three years, and often within months, whereas treatment increases the risk that they will spread.

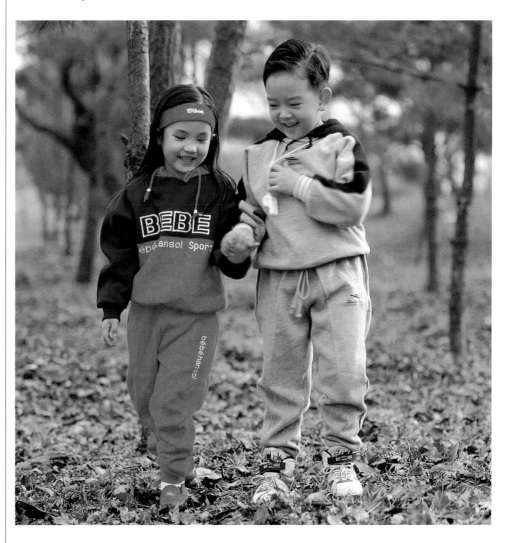

▲ *The virus that causes warts is contagious and can be passed on by holding hands with someone affected. This explains why children transmit it to each other.*

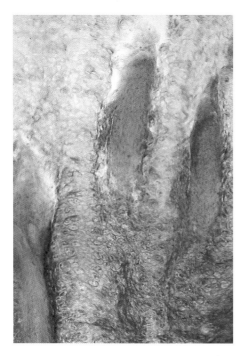

▲ *This photomicrograph of a slice of wart tissue shows the mass of active mutant cells (in purple) that are responsible for the growth of the wart.*

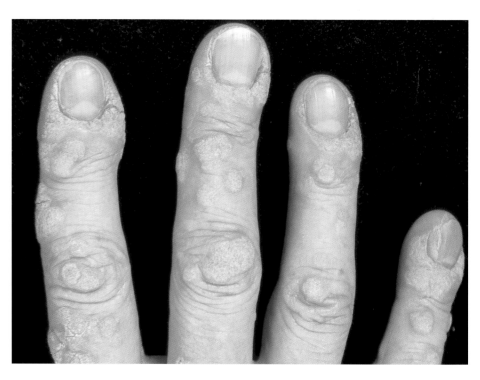

▲ *Clusters of warts on the hands can be unsightly and inhibiting. Either freezing or electrical burning techniques will remove them, in most cases, permanently. Sometimes they disappear spontaneously.*

proliferate in a disordered fashion, producing, in effect, a small, benign tumor. This is of interest to doctors, since warts are one of the few growths found in humans that are definitely known to be caused by a virus (see Growths).

The wart virus is contagious and can thus be transmitted from one person to another or from one part of the body to another,

▼ *Troublesome adult warts on the face can be irritating and are best removed, especially if they obstruct vision.*

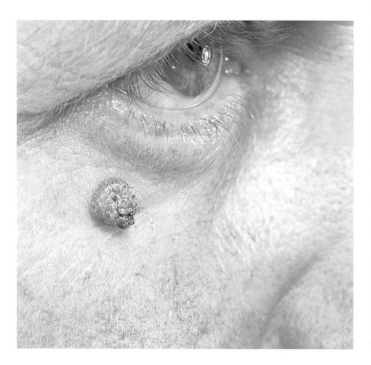

either by direct skin contact or indirectly by an intermediate object such as a towel. A break in the skin, such as a scratch, may facilitate entry of the virus.

Warts on the hand are most probably transmitted by hand-holding; genital warts are transmitted by sexual intercourse. The period between infection and the appearance of the warts may be weeks or months.

Warts on children are rarely transmitted to adults, probably because adults have acquired some immunity to the virus through infection during their own childhood. The viruses that cause common warts on the hand and genital warts are slightly different, so a person who was afflicted with hand warts during childhood is not immune to genital warts during adulthood.

Appearance

The appearance of warts varies a little according to where they occur on the body. Warts on the palms of the hands are usually solitary growths consisting of a hard, dome-shaped, raised area of skin with hundreds of tiny conical projections, which give the surface of the wart a velvetlike appearance.

The color of warts also varies from pink to brown. Warts on the hands, knees, or face are often numerous and sometimes have a flat, plateaulike surface. Another variety, called filiform warts, consists of fine, elongated outgrowths that appear on the face or neck.

Genital warts may occur in and around the folds of skin of the vulva in women or around the tip of the penis in men, or anywhere in the surrounding genital area. They often grow and spread profusely, creating clusters of cauliflower-like growths that, despite their rather unsightly appearance, cause little discomfort. Sometimes, however, they may obstruct normal sexual or excretory functions. The presence of genital warts should always be reported

"Magic" cures

The treatment of warts has a rich history of myth and magic, most of which probably originated in medieval days, when sufferers would have consulted the local healer for treatment. Herbs, chants, and incantations were the standard weapons against most ailments, and these treatments were effective in dealing with warts. Indeed, some of these methods are still used in rural districts. For no good medical reason, they sometimes appeared to have the desired result but it is probably more realistic to assume that the warts were about to disappear anyway.

However, some old wives' remedies may have some beneficial psychological effect, because if one is positively convinced that the remedy will work, then it is possible that this may promote the wart's disappearance.

Here are some improbable cures:

Tape a cat's hair to each wart

Rub the leaves of a plant called wartwort over the growth

Bury a piece of meat in the yard

Leave a bag of pebbles with a silver coin inside by the wayside; if the finder keeps the silver coin, he or she will get a wart, while the sufferer is cured

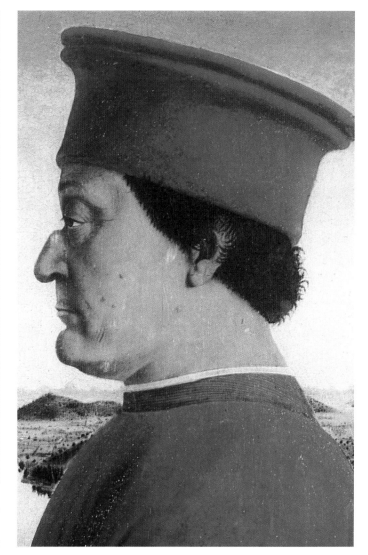

▲ *The famous Renaissance portrait of the duke of Urbino by Piero della Francesca is remarkable for its realism, showing hooked nose, warts and all.*

to a doctor, since they often accompany more serious sexually transmitted infections (see Sexually Transmitted Diseases).

All warts have tiny blood capillaries, and if the surface of the wart is cut away, these appear as tiny bleeding points, or as black seeds, on the surface of the wart where the blood in the capillaries has coagulated. The presence or absence of these bleeding points or black filaments helps doctors to distinguish warts from other skin growths of similar appearance.

Treatment

Over the centuries a wide variety of folk remedies have been used in the treatment of warts, ranging from chants and incantations to rubbing the warts with plants or vegetables. A number of people have also claimed that they have special gifts or talents for charming warts away. Some people claim that hypnosis works and the warts just disappear afterward. Although these unconventional cures may sometimes appear to work, a visit to the doctor will probably have a more rewarding result.

There are a number of more conventional treatments for warts, but there are no specific drugs for combating the wart virus. However, the growths can be attacked with corrosive ointments, or by freezing, scraping, or electrically burning them off. All of these procedures are carried out by a doctor.

Common childhood warts on the hands and knees can be left to disappear in their own time, or they can be treated painlessly with an antiseptic acid paint. Applied twice a day, this usually causes the wart to disappear in two or three months.

Troublesome adult warts on the face or hands are sometimes treated by freezing with liquid nitrogen or solid carbon dioxide, which can be mildly painful but is very effective and causes little scarring. Electrically burning a wart off is more likely to cause a scar and is often followed by a recurrence of the infection, so this technique is less often used.

Genital warts are treated either by surgery or topically by applying a corrosive substance, such as podophyllin. This must be applied by a doctor or nurse, since careless application of the ointment causes soreness. It is important to wash the ointment off some four to six hours after it has been applied. Podophyllin is never used to treat genital warts during pregnancy, since it may be absorbed into the body and can have harmful effects on the fetus.

However, even though a wart has disappeared or been permanently removed, the wart virus sometimes lies dormant in the skin and may resume its activity some weeks or even months later.

See also: **Side effects; Skin and skin diseases; Viruses**

Weight

Questions and Answers

I try to lose weight, with no success. Can my doctor give me drugs to stop me from overeating?

Weight loss involves balancing energy intake with energy use. In extreme cases, a doctor may give you appetite suppressing drugs, but many have side effects, including addiction. Increased exercise and cutting down high-calorie foods will help weight loss.

I have been very overweight for years. What should I do?

Surgery is possible in severe cases of obesity, but it is not always successful. The stomach can be stitched to reduce its size, however, nutritional advice should also be provided to prevent a relapse after surgery.

My daughter exercises too much and eats very little. How can I encourage her to increase her body weight?

She may have anorexia nervosa. It is an eating disorder that involves obsessive dieting, often accompanied by excessive exercise. Sufferers are usually obsessive in other ways as well, constantly cleaning and cooking for other members of the family, for example. They are often high achievers at school. The condition can have very harmful effects on the body and in some cases is fatal. It is essential to seek medical advice early if you suspect your daughter has anorexia nervosa. Your doctor will monitor her weight, and may advise counseling or other therapy. If you have difficulty in persuading your daughter to go to the doctor, try to find another pretext, such as brittle hair or a lack of periods (also symptoms of anorexia nervosa). Simply telling her to stop dieting and start exercising will not work. She needs professional help.

A person's weight in relation to his or her height is an indicator of fitness. For some people, weight watching is an obsession, whereas for others, food is an obsession; and the result is overweight and obesity.

To define overweight and obesity, desirable weight standards are calculated based on height and weight. The formula is known as body mass index (BMI). A BMI of 25 to 29.9 is considered overweight, whereas a BMI of 30 is considered obese. Statistics from 2001 showed that more than one in three people in the United States (37 percent) was overweight compared with 31 percent in 1990. The figures for obesity have nearly doubled over the same period—from 11 percent in 1990 to 21 percent in 2001. The problem is also increasing among children, and 15 percent of children between six and 19 are now overweight. In the late 1960s, this figure was between 4 and 5 percent. Children who are overweight are more likely to become obese in adult life.

Being overweight has been shown to increase the risk of death from a range of disorders, including high blood pressure; coronary heart disease; stroke; type II diabetes; gallbladder disease; osteoarthritis and respiratory disorders; and sleep apnea (cessation of breathing during sleep). Risks from certain cancers, including breast, prostate, and colon cancer are also greater in overweight people. Being underweight can also be bad for the health. Underweight people are prone to deficiencies of nutrients, anemia, osteoporosis, and heart problems (see Heart Attack).

Weight as a symptom of a disorder

Being underweight or overweight is not in itself an illness, but it may be a symptom of a disorder. Weight gain or weight loss, or both, may be a result of eating disorders and other psychological disorders such as depression (see Anorexia and Bulimia). Many people eat for comfort in times of stress; other people find it difficult to eat when they are anxious.

Sudden weight gain often occurs at puberty when changing hormone levels affect the bulk of muscle in teenage bodies and increase the level of fat stores, particularly in girls. Weight gain is also a symptom of pregnancy. Such changes are normal, but must not be excessive. Weight gain or loss is also associated with contraceptive pill use. New users should monitor weight, and

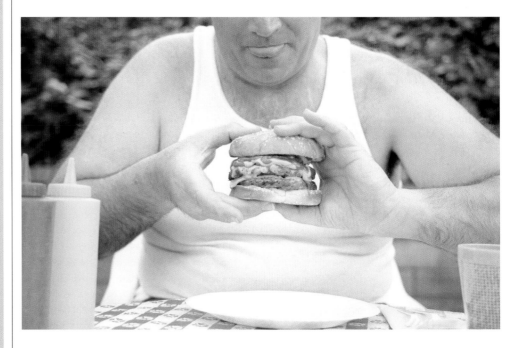

▲ *Taking little exercise, and getting into a habit of eating large meals that have a large amount of saturated fat, is a certain way to put on excess weight.*

BMI	20	22	24	26	28	30	32	34	36	38	40	42	44	46	48	50	52	53	54
Height (in.)	Body weight (lb.)																		
58	96	105	115	126	134	143	153	162	172	181	191	201	210	220	229	239	248	253	258
59	99	109	119	128	138	148	158	168	178	188	198	208	217	227	237	247	257	262	267
60	102	112	123	133	143	153	163	174	184	194	204	215	225	235	245	255	266	271	276
61	106	116	127	137	148	158	169	180	190	201	211	222	232	243	254	264	275	280	285
62	109	120	131	142	153	164	175	186	196	207	218	229	240	251	262	273	284	289	295
63	113	124	135	146	152	169	180	191	203	214	225	237	248	259	270	282	293	299	304
64	116	128	140	151	163	174	186	197	209	221	232	244	256	267	279	291	302	308	314
65	120	132	144	156	168	180	192	204	216	228	240	252	264	276	288	500	312	318	324
66	124	136	148	161	173	186	198	210	223	235	247	260	272	284	297	309	322	328	334
67	127	140	153	166	178	191	204	217	230	242	255	268	280	293	306	319	331	338	344
68	131	144	158	171	184	187	219	223	230	236	249	276	289	302	315	328	341	348	354
69	135	149	162	176	189	203	216	230	243	257	270	284	297	311	324	338	351	358	365
70	139	153	167	181	195	209	222	236	250	264	278	292	306	320	334	348	362	369	376
71	143	157	172	186	200	215	229	243	257	272	286	301	315	329	343	358	372	379	386
72	147	162	177	191	206	221	235	250	265	279	294	309	324	338	353	368	383	390	397
73	151	166	182	197	212	227	242	257	272	288	302	318	333	348	363	378	393	401	408
74	155	171	186	202	218	233	249	264	280	295	311	326	342	358	373	389	404	412	420
75	160	176	192	208	224	240	256	272	287	303	319	335	351	367	383	399	415	423	431

▲ *Find height in the left-hand column. Read across row to find weight. The figure at the top of this column is the BMI.*

consult their clinic if symptoms persist after a few months of use.

Weight gain may also be a symptom of edema—water retention, which can be caused by kidney and liver disorders. Edema can be treated by diuretic drugs prescribed by a doctor, but the underlying causes should be investigated and treated. Edema in pregnancy is a serious condition because it is one of the symptoms of the life-threatening disorder preeclampsia. Other symptoms are high blood pressure and protein in the urine. Regular checks for these symptoms are routine at prenatal clinics. Rest, and in severe cases, hospital bed rest, is the main form of treatment. Drugs to prevent convulsions may be prescribed, and early delivery may be necessary since the condition does not persist for long after labor.

Sudden weight loss may also be a symptom of an underlying disorder. If someone loses more than 10 pounds over a period of 10 weeks without being on a weight-reduction diet or taking increased exercise, he or she should check for other symptoms that might indicate a problem.

Unexplained weight loss

If weight loss is accompanied by a feeling of restlessness, sweating, weakness, and difficulty sleeping, the problem may be an overactive thyroid gland. If weight loss is accompanied by excessive thirst, a need to urinate frequently, and general tiredness, the cause may be diabetes or another hormone deficiency. Weight loss with persistent diarrhea may be a symptom of a disorder in the digestive tract, which prevents absorption of food. Any unusual bowel habits, such

---

Calculating BMI

To calculate a child's BMI divide weight (in kilograms) by height x height (in meters).

$$BMI = \frac{weight\ (kg)}{height\ (m) \times height\ (m)}$$

If the metric equivalents are not known:

$$BMI = \frac{weight\ (lb.) \times 705}{height\ (in.) \times height\ (in.)}$$

Weil's disease

My wife is a veterinary surgeon and mentions Weil's disease, but sometimes calls it leptospirosis. Is there a difference?

Leptospirosis is a general term for infections caused by a spiral-shaped germ *Leptospira interrogans*. These infections vary in severity; some cause no symptoms at all, but some can be quite serious, even dangerous. Cases in which there is obvious illness with fever and jaundice are usually called Weil's disease. In 90 percent of cases there is no jaundice and these cases almost always have milder symptoms.

My husband recently had Weil's disease and I discovered that the disease is caused by a spirochete. I understand that spirochetes cause syphilis. Will I be at risk of getting syphilis?

No. There are many different spirochete germs and the one that causes Weil's disease, *Leptospira interrogans*, is a different organism from *Treponema pallidum*, which causes syphilis. They are both spirochaetes, but that describes their general shape. *Leptospira interrogans* cannot cause syphilis.

My son works in sewers. I know he wears protective clothing but I'm worried he might get Weil's disease. Is there a vaccine for it?

There are so many different strains (serotypes) of *Leptospira interrogans* that it is impracticable to produce a vaccine that protects against them all. Vaccines can be produced against particular strains if the type is prevalent in a local area. If the risk is considered high an antibiotic can be taken weekly for a time. And in the event of direct contact with water known to be contaminated with the germ, preventive antibiotics can be given.

This potentially dangerous disease is transmitted in the urine of rats, dogs, and many other small mammals. The risk of infection is small except in people whose employment brings them into contact with rats.

Weil's disease most often affects farm-workers, people working with animals, and those who frequently comes in contact with rat-infected wet areas. It was formerly a serious hazard to sewer workers, canal workers, miners, and people employed in fish markets. Awareness of the risks and improvements in working conditions have greatly reduced the incidence of the disease.

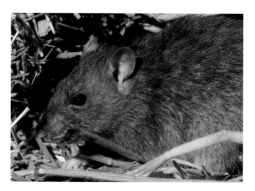

▲ *Rats are often infected with the spirochete that causes Weil's disease.*

Cause and symptoms

The disease is an infection caused by a spiral-shaped germ called *Leptospira interrogans*. It is usually acquired by contact with water contaminated with the urine of dogs, rodents, and other wild animals that are infected with the spirochete. The germ penetrates through abrasions in the skin or through the intact mucous membranes of the eyes, nose, or vagina. Prolonged contact with water containing the germs may even allow infection to penetrate intact skin. Infection is also possible through the intestine if food contaminated with leptospirae has been eaten.

The disease usually starts seven to 12 days after infection, but the incubation period may range from two to 20 days. Symptoms are very general because the germs quickly spread to every part of the body. There is intense, throbbing headache, with severe pain and tenderness in the muscles, fever, shivering, joint and bone pain, sore throat, and cough. The liver is enlarged and frequently the spleen and the lymph nodes are also swollen.

The nervous system is typically involved and in some cases this may lead to mental disturbances including delirium, hallucination, and even psychotic behavior. Irregularities of the heartbeat are common. Possible complications include heart failure, meningitis, internal eye inflammation (uveitis), kidney failure, neuritis, nerve paralyses, and Guillain-Barré syndrome (see Guillain-Barré Syndrome). The jaundice, which is caused by liver damage, may last from a few days to several weeks.

Diagnosis and treatment

Weil's disease must be distinguished from other illnesses such as glandular fever, dengue fever, malaria, brucellosis, hepatitis, typhoid, relapsing fever, pneumonia, and viral meningitis. Unless there is a history of contact with water likely to be contaminated with rat's urine, Weil's disease may not be suspected.

There is an antibody test that is rapid and easy, but the presence of antibodies does not necessarily imply a current infection. If repeated antibody checks show a sharp rise in the levels of antibodies, however, the diagnosis of Weil's disease is highly likely. The causal germs can be cultured from the blood early in the infection.

The germs are susceptible to a range of antibiotics including penicillin, streptomycin, tetracycline, and erythromycin. To be effective, antibiotics must be given within four to seven days of the onset of the disease. Care and close observation are required, because the rapid killing of the germs may cause an acute, and sometimes dangerous, allergic reaction to the released bacterial material.

> *See also:* Infection and infectious diseases; Meningitis; Typhoid and paratyphoid

Wellness

Questions and Answers

Does being thin equal wellness?

An obsessive interest in thinness is not healthy and may lead to a person's needing help from a doctor, nutritional therapist, or psychotherapist. Over time, a well-balanced diet and moderate regular exercise will help weight problems. Dieting can result in the loss of healthy tissue as well as fat; metabolism slows down, thereby counteracting the effect of reduced food intake. You must change your habits permanently. Fashionable thinness is not the same as healthy thinness.

Do you have to abstain from alcohol, coffee, and cigarettes completely to be well?

Holistic practitioners advise cutting these substantially, since they unbalance the system. Doctors advise women to drink fewer than 14 units of alcohol a week and men fewer than 21 units. One unit equals a glass of wine, a shot of liquor, or a bottle of beer. Some wine may actually help to keep heart disease at bay. Up to three cups of coffee or tea a day are unlikely to do harm. As for smoking, this is recognized as the single most avoidable risk factor for ill-health. There are no valid arguments to justify smoking.

Can you be well if you have a disability or have a chronic illness?

Wellness is being as well as possible given our circumstances. A healthy diet is even more important for people who are already struggling with illness. People with disabilities can use specially designed exercise programs. Holistic medicine is ideal for improving the quality of life for people for whom doctors can do little: for example, massage for pain, and hypnotherapy for depression.

Is wellness more than just absence of illness and, if so, how can it be achieved? Many people are free from serious problems, but frequently suffer symptoms such as headaches and sleeplessness.

Because there is so much conflicting advice about how to stay healthy, the pursuit of health can seem complicated. We are led to believe that perfect health is within everyone's reach, so that, if we are sick, we find it all too easy to blame ourselves: we have not relaxed enough, we have not exercised enough, or we have eaten and drunk the wrong things. The best orthodox doctors understand that good medicine is holistic medicine and that patients are more than mere cases.

If someone wishes to try alternative or complementary medicine, more choices and research are required to decide on the best and most appropriate therapy.

Conventional medicine, provided by doctors and hospitals, takes a different view of illness and wellness from alternative medicine (see Holistic Medicine). Not all doctors take the view that if there is nothing seriously wrong, a patient is well. There are doctors who have adopted a

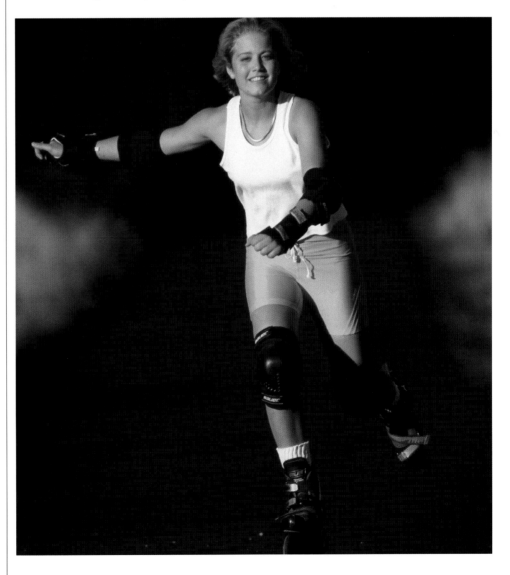

▲ *A good diet and plenty of exercise are not just about health in its purely physiological sense; health is also a joyous attitude to life.*

The healthy diet

Starchy foods—About half of what people eat should come from this group, which includes foods such as bread, rice, pasta, and potatoes. These are filling foods that are slowly absorbed. Whole-grain bread and brown rice and pasta are best from a nutritional point of view. This is because the outer layer of the grains contains all the vitamins and minerals and provides the fiber that maintains healthy digestion. The inner white part of the grain is just starch.

Fruit and vegetables—These are the antiaging and antisickness agents in our diet, and are probably the most vital part of it. According to the World Health Organization (WHO) we should have at least five servings of fruit and vegetables a day. Freshness and variety are important, as is the method of preparation. Vegetable should be scrubbed rather than peeled, and cooked for the minimum of time or, better still, eaten raw. Stir-frying, steaming, or stewing are better methods than boiling, in which some vitamins are lost in the cooking water.

Protein and fat—Adults do not have to eat protein at every meal. Only 10–15 percent of the diet needs to be made up of protein, and legumes, seeds, nuts, and grains (rice, wheat, and corn) can provide enough. Meat and dairy products should be cut down because they have a high saturated fat content and are not easily digested. Oily fish or flax oil is a rich source of omega-3 fatty acids.

Sugary foods—Sugar and sugary foods such as carbonated drinks, candy, desserts, cookies, and cakes provide quick calories and few vitamins. Sugar is quickly digested and causes rapid fluctuations in our blood sugar levels. Sugary foods are tasty but they are not essential to the diet. They discourage the intake of healthier food with slow-release carbohydrates, such as that in fruit and vegetables, and those with a high-fiber content. Sugar and sugary foods are best kept to a minimum or avoided.

A healthy way of life

How many of these statements are true for you?

My health is good. I am about the right weight for my build and height. I give and receive affection. I express my feelings when angry or worried. I have fewer than three caffeine-containing drinks (coffee, cocoa, or cola) a day. I take part in regular social activities. I eat at least one full, well-balanced meal a day. I do something just for pleasure at least once a week. There is at least one relative within 50 miles of home on whom I can rely. I have some time alone during the day. I get seven or eight hours of sleep at least four nights a week. I exercise hard enough to work up a sweat at least twice a week. I have a network of friends and acquaintances. I discuss problems such as work and money with other members of the household. I have at least one friend I can talk to about personal affairs. I would never consider smoking cigarettes. I organize my time well. I have fewer than five alcoholic drinks a week.

mechanistic form of practice in which only the presenting symptoms are considered and the only treatment given is drug treatment. Often, unlike alternative medical practitioners, orthodox doctors are too busy to engage in fully holistic consultations. This is regrettable, since many people believe that human interactions in medicine are important.

Holistic medicine sees people as a whole—body, mind, emotions, and spirit. If all these parts are functioning properly and in harmony, people have a built-in ability to heal themselves and cope with external stresses (see Stress), whether caused by germs, the weather (see Seasonal Affective Disorder), bereavement (see Grief), and so on. The desired state for humans is health and happiness.

The function of holistic therapies is preventive as much as curative. With regard to maintaining health from day to day, doctors tend to lay down general rules, whereas holistic practitioners feel that everyone has to find his or her own way of achieving health. The main goal is to work within individual limitations, to find a balanced way of life. Both doctors and holistic practitioners, however, agree that the basis of health is knowledge, diet, exercise, and relaxation. Holistic practitioners go further and say that these are fundamental to our well-being.

Diet

There is no single diet that suits everyone. Personal preferences and dietary restrictions caused by health conditions must be taken into consideration. For example, people who are very active or women who are pregnant or breast-feeding require more protein. People have different dietary needs according to their body type, where

they live, and even the seasons. There may be practical, physical, or psychological reasons that make it difficult for people to eat in a balanced way. Lack of money and time can make it difficult to eat fresh food and have regular meals. It is very common for people to crave the very food that is worst for them, and many physical illnesses (see Irritable Bowel Syndrome) and even psychological ones (see Anorexia and Bulimia) may be caused by the wrong diet or nutritional deficiencies (see Vitamins). Emotional problems can lead to erratic eating, over- and undereating, or eating the wrong foods for comfort. However, there are some basic guidelines that are relevant to everyone. A typical Western diet is associated with diabetes, obesity, heart disease, and strokes, largely owing to too much sugar, saturated fat, refined foods, and alcohol. Instead, what is better is a good intake of fresh vegetables and fruit; dietary fiber in the form of whole grains, nuts, and legumes; less meat and dairy products; less sugar; and avoidance of processed foods.

Exercise

People need to exercise (see Exercise) at least two or three times a week for 45 to 60 minutes to keep their body in good working order. Short, regular sessions are better and there is less chance of injury than with sporadic, prolonged sessions.

Not only does exercise keep people fit; it also can make them feel better emotionally and psychologically. Medical research in the United States has shown that it can be as effective as psychotherapy (see Psychotherapy) in treating depression (see Depression). Exercises such as yoga (see Yoga) and tai chi (see Tai Chi) work on the body's subtle energy, which is thought to flow around the body.

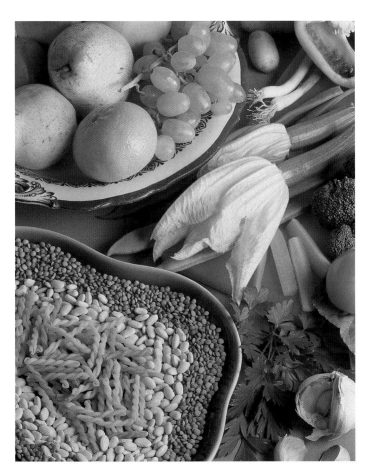

Just as with the circulation of the blood (see Circulatory System), energy flow can become uneven and even blocked, and exercise is designed to rebalance and free it. Acupuncture (see Acupuncture), acupressure, shiatsu (see Shiatsu), and reflexology (see Reflexology) are claimed to work with the same energy. After this type of exercise people should feel both calmer and more full of vitality.

Relaxation and stress management

Stress (see Stress; Stress Management) is caused by a failure to deal with the problems that face us. Even happy events, such as the birth of a baby, can cause stress because of lifestyle changes.

There is no doubt that some illness is stress-related. Stress can, rarely, lead to a weakening of the immune system (see Immune System) and make people more vulnerable to certain illnesses. When people are stressed they are tense, and tension leads to soreness and even serious problems in internal organs. Relaxation (see Relaxation) is one of the most important ways of coping with stress. Everyone has his or her own way of relaxing, whether it is painting, listening to music, going for a walk, or doing something for someone else. Physical relaxation helps prevent habitual bad posture (see Posture) such as hunched shoulders, which lead to aches and pains. Yoga classes always end with the corpse posture for physical and mental relaxation. The Alexander technique (see Alexander Technique) can also help with physical relaxation. If people find it difficult to relax, learning meditation techniques (see Meditation), autogenic training, or even self-hypnosis (see Hypnosis) can help. Counseling and psychotherapy can teach people to react better to stressful situations or help them to find purpose in their lives. They can also help with unresolved conflicts.

◄ *Ensuring a good intake of plenty of fresh fruits and vegetables, particularly green leafy vegetables, rather than relying on ready-prepared or processed foods, can contribute to health and a sense of well-being.*

Exercise and what it can do

Exercise helps maintain a correct weight. Aerobic exercise is activity that increases the body's demand for oxygen, speeds up the metabolism, and uses up extra calories. It improves the function of the lungs and heart so that the whole body is nourished by oxygen and blood. There are different ways to do this, such as climbing stairs, fast walking, jogging, team sports, bicycling, and swimming. Exercise builds up strength. Strong muscles maintain bones in position so that common orthopedic disorders are avoided. Strong muscles are also less likely to be injured. Backache is often caused by strained muscles and poor posture, which causes the vertebrae to press on nerves. Keeping fit, gymnastic workouts, climbing, aikido, and some types of dance can all increase strength. Certain types of exercise keep people supple. Suppleness is having joints that work fully so that people can bend and stretch and move easily without pain. Decreasing suppleness happens during the aging process. Dance, yoga, or tai chi increases suppleness. These types of exercise are ideal for older people, or for people unused to exercise, because they are gentle and noncompetitive.

A definition of wellness

The following definition of wellness comes from George Ohsawa, the founder of macrobiotics (see Macrobiotics), a dietary system based on traditional Japanese teachings. He lists the following seven conditions for true wellness:

Never being tired. If we feel tired it is because we are not resting properly, change our minds too much, or are not flexible enough to cope with our changing circumstances.

Having a good appetite—for food, sex, work, knowledge, experience, happiness, health, and life. Oversatisfaction reduces our appetite, so we should aim always to be slightly hungry and keep emptiness within ourselves.

Sleeping well. This means sleeping deeply, not sleeping a long time, and is the result of energetic physical and mental activity while we are awake. Restless sleep is due to mental unrest.

Having a good memory. This enables us to be wise. The healthier we become the more we remember, till we remember our true origins and become aware of our spiritual destiny.

Never being angry. If we are truly healthy, we are in harmony with our environment. Health is the capacity to accept all circumstances with a smile and change difficulties into opportunities.

Being joyous and alert. Joyousness is a natural result of good health and eating well day to day.

Having endless appreciation. Even when we are physically sick, we are healthy if we are aware that we are the cause of our own sickness, are thankful for the opportunity to learn, and surrender our destiny to nature in a spirit of endless appreciation.

Conversely, we may be without physical or mental symptoms of disease, but unless a deep gratitude permeates our whole life, we are not truly healthy and whole.

See also: **Alternative medicine**

West Nile virus

Questions and Answers

I heard that West Nile virus is an arbovirus. What is this?

The term "arbovirus" does not refer to a particular kind of virus. It refers to any of the viruses spread by blood-feeding insects such as mosquitos, sandflies, and ticks. About 100 of these viruses can cause disease in humans. "Arbovirus" is a contraction of "arthropod-borne" and an arthropod is any jointed-legged animal such as an insect, spider, tick, centipede, or millipede. The arthropods form the largest phylum in the whole animal kingdom. The West Nile virus is transmitted by mosquitos.

Is it true that West Nile virus can affect the brain?

Yes. Although most people affected suffer only a very mild and brief illness, a proportion develop brain inflammation (encephalitis) or meningitis (inflammation of the brain coverings). This complication occurs rarely in young people, but in the older age groups it carries a death rate of about 9 percent.

Did West Nile virus infection occur owing to organ transplantation?

Yes. Four organs taken from a deceased donor caused West Nile virus infection in the four recipients. It has also occurred in laboratory workers handling the brains of dead birds.

I have read that the West Nile virus is a flavivirus. What is this?

The flaviviruses are a genus of arboviruses that include viruses that cause yellow fever, St. Louis encephalitis, and dengue fever. The first to be discovered was the yellow fever virus. "Flavus" is a Latin word for yellow so it became the generic name for these viruses.

West Nile virus was first recognized in the Western Hemisphere in an outbreak in New York in August 1999. Since then thousands of people have been infected, and some of the older victims have died.

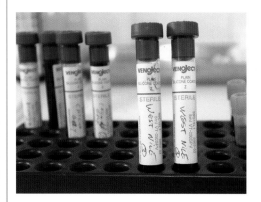

▲ *Blood samples of horses suspected of having West Nile virus.*

West Nile virus was first identified in a human patient in Uganda in 1937, but it was not until August 1999 that it was detected as a cause of human disease in the United States. An investigation of brain inflammation (encephalitis) in two patients in Queens, New York, showed that this virus was the cause. The virus then spread westward until by the end of 2002 well over 3,000 people had been infected and the disease was occurring in all but seven states of the Union.

Of all those infected 69 percent developed encephalitis or meningitis, and in this group 199 people died. The middle value (median) age of those who died was 78 and deaths were not necessarily caused exclusively by the virus. The older the patient, the more likely the outcome was to be fatal (see Encephalitis).

The West Nile virus is very similar to the virus that caused the epidemic of St. Louis encephalitis in which 2,100 cases occurred, with 170 deaths (8 percent). Both conditions are spread by culex mosquitos and in both cases birds, especially crows and blue jays, are involved as intermediate hosts for the virus. In 2002, the number of counties reporting dead birds infected with West Nile virus was five times higher than in 2001. During the same period the number of reported cases of this infection in horses rose twelvefold. Only about a third of people infected recall having been bitten by a mosquito in the month prior to the onset of the disease.

West Nile virus belongs to a virus group known as the flaviviruses that includes those causing St. Louis encephalitis, Kunjin and Murray Valley encephalitis, and Japanese encephalitis. The virus is extensively present in wild and domestic birds in Africa, Asia, and Europe. The outbreak in New York in 1999 was the first sign of this infection in the Western world.

Symptoms and diagnosis

Illness from this virus is essentially a disease of the elderly. Although it may occur in people of all ages from five to 90, the great majority (88 percent) are 50 years of age or over. The illness presents as fever with hot flashes, night sweats, weakness, nausea, and vomiting. About one in five infected persons has a measleslike rash on some part of the skin. If headache, stiff neck, bladder dysfunction, alteration in mental state, and respiratory distress occur, the implication is that encephalitis has developed. This complication occurs in roughly half the cases. Spinal cord involvement causing poliomyelitis is another possible complication.

The diagnosis of West Nile virus infection can be made by culture of the virus from the blood, by the finding of specific antibodies to the virus, and by finding the RNA of the virus in tissue samples. These tests will be done if suspicion of the diagnosis is raised by clinical symptoms and signs occurring in the presence of an epidemic of the disease.

Treatment

In the great majority of cases the disease is self-limiting and the viruses are dealt with by the antibodies they provoke. When encephalitis or meningitis develops, treatment with immune globulin and general supportive measures may be necessary.

See also: **Meningitis; Viruses**

Wheezing

What actually causes the sound of wheezing?

It is produced by air being forced through narrow tubes (bronchi) in the lungs. It can be high- or low-pitched, and works on the same principle as a wind instrument: the narrower the tube, the higher the note. If a single bronchus is narrowed, a single wheeze is produced, but many different-sized bronchi may be affected, causing many simultaneous notes.

If I wheeze, should I quit smoking?

Yes. Cigarette smoke is an irritant and will make wheezing worse. Smoking can cause chronic bronchitis leading to permanent narrowing of the bronchi.

Is the wheezing caused by asthma permanent?

No. Many asthmatics are entirely normal between attacks, but they require regular treatment to prevent further attacks.

Is wheezing always a symptom of disease, or can it occur on its own?

Wheezing can be a normal reflex. If someone is exposed to toxic fumes or dust, a reflex bronchospasm may result: this is an attempt by the body to protect the lungs from further damage.

After a heart attack, my husband wakes at night wheezing and breathless. Why?

It is likely that he is suffering from episodes of pulmonary edema. When a person is lying flat, fluid tends to accumulate in the lungs more easily. Sleeping with three or four pillows may alleviate these symptoms, but he should see his doctor and ask him or her to review his treatment.

The sound of wheezing is unmistakable—and sometimes frightening. Depending on the cause, it can be mild or severe, with or without recurrent episodes. However, treatment can do much to alleviate symptoms.

Wheezing occurs when the normal flow of air into and out of the lungs during breathing is partially obstructed by a narrowing of the airways. The noise produced is more marked during breathing out, when the air is being forced out of the lungs against the bronchial obstruction.

Mechanism

Narrowing of a bronchus may be caused by spasm of the muscle that lines the bronchi, for example, in asthma; excessive production of mucus by the glands in the bronchial wall causing infection or chronic bronchitis; or edema: that is, fluid produced by inflammation or by heart

CAUSES OF WHEEZING

Interference with the passage of air into and out of the lungs produces wheezing. The lung section (bottom right) illustrates how, in pulmonary edema, excess fluid between air sacs cuts down the amount of oxygen that passes into the bloodstream. The other diagrams show cross sections of bronchi with various causes of obstruction.

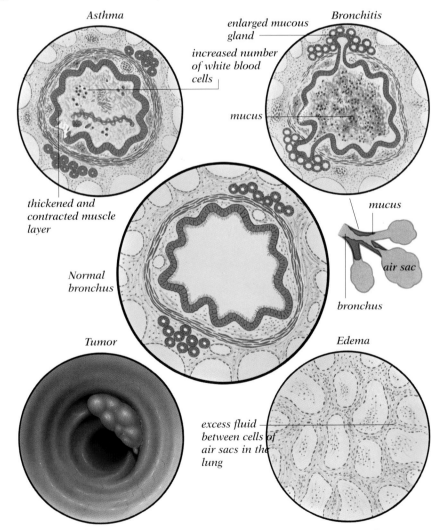

Asthma

enlarged mucous gland

increased number of white blood cells

Bronchitis

mucus

thickened and contracted muscle layer

mucus

air sac

Normal bronchus

bronchus

Tumor

Edema

excess fluid between cells of air sacs in the lung

failure. Often a combination of these conditions is involved. In time this may lead to widespread narrowing of many airways (bronchi), which can have serious effects on the function of the lungs. Occasionally a single bronchus may be narrowed, for example, by an inhaled foreign body or by a tumor growing into the bronchus.

Causes

In asthma, which is the most common cause of narrowed bronchi, the symptoms are attacks of breathlessness and wheezing, which can last from a few minutes to several hours or even days (see Asthma) and they are recurrent. The attacks are often precipitated by trigger factors such as allergy, infection, stress, or exercise.

Acute bronchitis (infection of the bronchi) can cause excessive amounts of mucus to be produced and may also cause wheezing (see Bronchitis). Acute bronchitis is much less common in babies and young children, and it causes only mild wheezing in these cases. Chronic bronchitis can also cause wheezing because the damaged airways are already narrowed. As with asthma, factors such as infection, strenuous exercise, or cigarette smoking may precipitate or increase the wheezing attacks.

▲ *The area around the Moskva River in Moscow, Russia, is so polluted with thick smoke that visibility is reduced and visitors have to wear masks.*

Sudden attacks of breathlessness and wheezing can sometimes occur in a person suffering from heart disease or following a heart attack, and are due to a different mechanism. If the heart is not functioning normally it may be unable to pump blood through the lungs efficiently, leading to the accumulation of fluid in the lungs (pulmonary edema). In such a case, the wheezing may be accompanied by chest pain (see Edema). Urgent medical treatment and usually hospitalization are required without delay.

Diagnosis

Diagnosis is made by assessing the factors that have contributed to an attack, and the degree of airway obstruction. This is done by using a flowmeter (which measures the speed at which the air can be blown out of the lungs) and a vitallograph (which measures the volume of air blown out over a given time). From the results an assessment can be made of how much of the airways' narrowing is reversible with treatment, and how much is irreversible owing to permanent damage to the bronchi.

Treatment

Treatment will depend on the outcome of the investigation to discover the cause of the wheezing, and the severity and frequency of the attacks. An isolated attack brought on by acute bronchitis is usually mild and resolves itself quickly. Infection requires treatment with antibiotics and possibly a cough expectorant.

If the wheezing is severe, a bronchodilator such as ventolin may be given, either as an aerosol or in tablet form.

When there is recurrent wheezing from asthma or chronic bronchitis, regular treatment is necessary using bronchodilators and other drugs to ensure that the airways are kept open. Drugs are usually administered as pills, which may be given as a long-acting preparation that need be taken only once or twice daily, or by inhalers. For asthma sufferers, preventive treatment is also given using intal or becotide inhalers, and it is important that these are used regularly even when the patient feels well.

A sudden, severe attack of wheezing is usually due to acute asthma or acute pulmonary edema and requires urgent medical treatment. If a known asthmatic does become wheezy, two or three extra puffs of his or her inhaler may avert the attack. However, if wheezing persists, medical help should be promptly sought. An appropriate treatment is to change the inhaler medication or administer injections of rapid-acting bronchodilators to the patient.

Acute pulmonary edema requires urgent treatment in a hospital, life-supportive measures such as high-concentration oxygen, intravenous diuretics to relieve the lungs of the excess fluid, morphine, intravenous bronchodilators, and sometimes bleeding to reduce venous return to the lungs.

Outlook

In general, the treatment for wheezing is very effective. In the majority of asthmatics the narrowing of the bronchi can be reversed completely to normal between attacks; but when a patient is suffering from more severe asthma or chronic bronchitis, the narrowing may be only partially reversible.

However, while wheezing and breathlessness can be extremely disabling, modern medical treatment has much to offer to alleviate uncomfortable symptoms (see Symptoms).

See also: **Allergies; Exercise**

Whiplash injury

Questions and Answers

Will wearing a seat belt prevent a whiplash injury?

No. The injury occurs when the head snaps back suddenly if a vehicle is struck from behind. Properly adjusted headrests can prevent most of these injuries. Seat belts may lessen the severity of the injury by preventing the wearer from bouncing forward again once the initial blow is over, and may prevent other injuries when a driver or passenger could be flung against a windshield.

Is it true that a whiplash injury can occur when a baby is abused?

It is possible for a whiplash injury to occur in these circumstances. It may, however, be much more difficult to diagnose than more obvious injuries caused by child abuse because there are usually no outward signs of injury at all. Because a baby cannot complain, especially of neck pain, such an injury might never be detected.

Are whiplash injuries as common today as they were 20 years ago?

Whiplash injuries have become more common over the past 20 years. This may be partly due to the increased number of vehicles on the road, but may also reflect an increasing tendency for victims to file for damages, so that more cases come to public attention.

Is it possible to break your neck in a whiplash injury?

It is rare for the bones of the neck to fracture in a whiplash injury. In a whiplash injury the head is jerked back and the soft tissues of the neck are sprained. Broken bones in the neck are caused when the neck is loaded by an abnormal weight—for example, when diving into shallow water and cracking the head on the bottom.

With more vehicles on the road than ever before, the chances of a whiplash injury, or a sprained neck, have increased. How should a whiplash be treated, and are there any measures that prevent it from occurring?

The term "whiplash injury" conjures up images of devastating damage to the neck. In fact, whiplash refers to a single type of neck injury that is essentially a sprain (see Sprains). Like any sprain, it can vary greatly in severity, ranging from a few days of mild discomfort to months of pain, or even to permanent disability. In the majority of cases, however, recovery is complete within about a month.

Causes

Whiplash injury is nearly always caused by traffic accidents, usually when a stationary automobile is struck from behind by another moving vehicle. When this happens, the occupants of the stationary automobile are suddenly propelled forward, causing their heads to be momentarily left behind. The neck is bent violently backward, and the muscles and ligaments at the front of the neck and throat are placed under a sudden strain. This results in minor hemorrhage (see Hemorrhage) into these muscles and ligaments, which resolves within a short period of time. In severe cases there may be momentary dislocation (see Dislocation) of one or

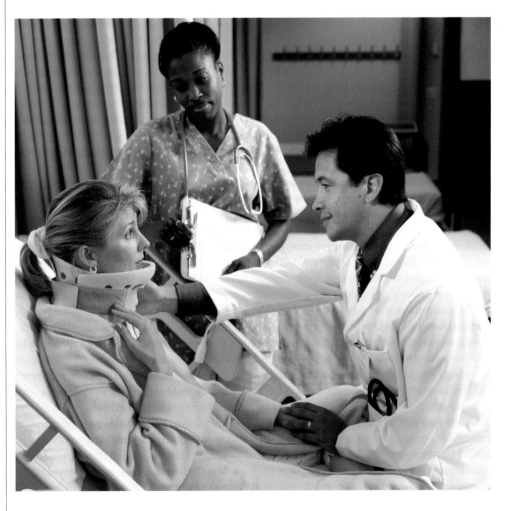

▲ *When a whiplash injury causes pain and stiffness, a neck brace supports the neck and allows the injured muscles time to recover.*

Whooping cough

Highly infectious and very distressing for sufferers, whooping cough can be one of childhood's most dangerous illnesses. However, it can be effectively prevented by immunization in infancy.

Whooping cough, or pertussis as it is medically known, is a highly infectious bacterial disease caused by *Bordetella pertussis*. Anybody who has neither had, nor been immunized against, whooping cough can catch it. The disease is spread by droplets of bacteria that are in the air. The bacteria settle in the mucous lining of the respiratory tract, causing inflammation and production of a thick, sticky mucus (see Bacteria; Inflammation; Mucus).

Symptoms of whooping cough and their incidence

Whooping cough in the unprotected may be severe and dangerous, especially in very young children, and often requires admission to the hospital. Nearly half of infants under one year who develop whooping cough suffer periods of failure of breathing, and about a quarter of those under six months of age show pneumonia on X-ray examination (see Breathing; Pneumonia). About 2 percent of all people with whooping cough suffer seizures, especially infants under six months. Out of 7,580 cases of whooping cough in the year 2001, there were 17 deaths, most of which occurred in babies younger than six months. The principal causes of death are brain damage from lack of oxygen, toxin from the *Bordetella* organism, and secondary bacterial infection (see Brain Damage and Disease; Infection and Infectious Diseases). Many babies are infected with whooping cough by adults who are suffering from a mild form of the disease, and whose earlier immunity has waned.

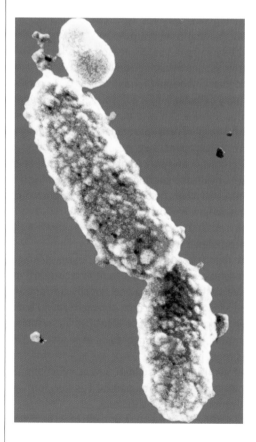

▲ *A scanning electron micrograph (SEM) of* Bordetella pertussis—*the bacterium that causes whooping cough.*

Course of the illness

The incubation period lasts six to 20 days from contact, with seven days as an average. The patient is infectious from the catarrhal phase and for about four weeks, and he or she should be isolated for a month or until the cough has stopped. Children under the age of one year in particular should be kept away from those who have the condition. The illness can be divided into three distinct stages: the catarrhal phase, the paroxysmal phase, and the convalescent phase.

The catarrhal phase lasts one or two weeks. Initially, the symptoms are rather like a cold: runny nose, red runny eyes, a slight cough, and fever (see Common Cold). The paroxysmal phase lasts from two to four or more weeks, and in this stage there are episodes of coughing, becoming increasingly worse and more frequent, often up to around 40 bouts a day. The bouts consist of five to 10 quickly repeated coughs while breathing out, followed by a prolonged effort to breathe in, which in older children produces the characteristic whoop. The face turns red or blue, the eyes bulge, the tongue sticks out, both eyes and nose run, and the veins in the neck become more obvious. Episodes of this coughing occur until the patient manages to dislodge the plug of mucus. During this time, in severe attacks, young children may lack oxygen and stop breathing or have a convulsion (see Convulsions; Oxygen).

At the end of the coughing bout the child will vomit. The vomiting is really more characteristic of whooping cough than the whoop. These episodes are extremely exhausting, and infants become tired and lose weight. Attacks can be triggered by movement, yawning, sneezing, eating, or drinking, or even by thinking about them. Between attacks, the patient appears relatively well.

During convalescence, the paroxysmal coughing, whooping, and vomiting gradually subside, although the cough and whoop may last for many weeks or months and they often recur if the child catches a cold or throat infection (see Throat).

Diagnosis

The diagnosis is usually made on the clinical symptoms, but in older children and adults who suffer a milder attack this can be difficult. The best method is to take a swab from the back of the nose and do a culture. Blood tests are not very helpful, though the number of lymphocytes (a type of defensive blood cell) may be very high, aiding diagnosis (see Lymphocytes). Otherwise, two samples of blood are needed, at the beginning and end of the illness, to show a rise in pertussis antibodies during that time. If the sample is not taken early enough, it will not show a large enough rise to make the diagnosis.

Complications

Most deaths from whooping cough are caused by complications such as pneumonia and brain damage. Usually pneumonia is due

▼ *These are some of the most common vaccines, including the DPT vaccine Infanrix (right), which is used to immunize against diphtheria, tetanus, and pertussis (whooping cough).*

not to pertussis bacteria, but to other invading bacteria that enter the affected lungs. Plugs of mucus may block off the bronchi (the tubes leading the air from the throat to the lungs), and cause the lung to collapse. It may then become infected by bacteria. Sometimes the lung collapse is permanent.

The most serious complications of the established disease in children who have not been protected by immunization are those affecting the brain. It must be remembered that the type of cough produced by this organism makes it almost impossible for the child to take a breath in the course of a paroxysm of coughing. One cough follows another so rapidly that there is not time to breathe in. It is only when the long paroxysm has passed that the child can inspire, and even then, obstruction to inspiration—the cause of the whoop—further impedes air intake. The thick mucus that forms in the bronchial tubes in whooping cough tends to obstruct the bronchi.

All this adds up to the risk that the child will fail to get enough oxygen. Since the brain has much higher oxygen requirements than any other organ of the body, this situation can lead to oxygen deprivation and brain damage. Although this is very rare, the effects can be disastrous. They include convulsions, blindness, deafness, movement disorders, paralysis, coma, and death.

Treatment

Antibiotics are not helpful once the illness has begun, but if the antibiotic erythromycin is given to a child who has been in contact with the disease before any symptoms appear, the severity of the illness may be reduced. The drug is given to children who have whooping cough because it makes these children less infectious to others (see Antibiotics).

Other treatment is symptomatic: avoiding stimuli that cause coughing; a warm room, especially at night; small and frequent

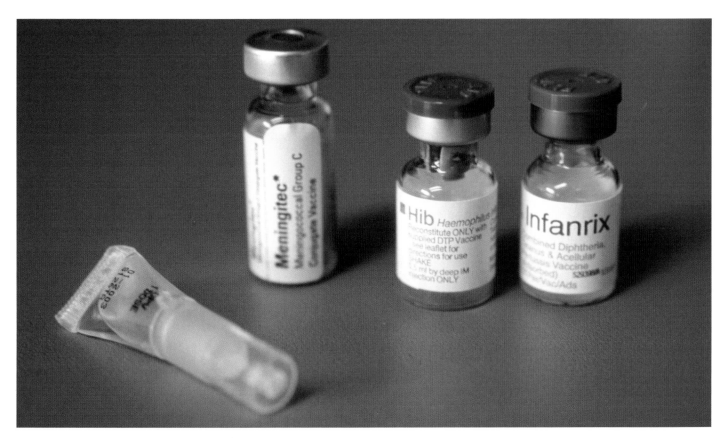

Questions and Answers

My daughter had whooping cough. Since then, she has had a series of coughs and colds. Is this because the illness has weakened her resistance to infection?

No. It's probably just bad luck. However, you should ask your doctor to check her over because sometimes part of the lung collapses after whooping cough and this may be her problem.

Is croup the same as whooping cough?

No. Croup arises from a viral infection that causes swelling of the larynx, so that when a child breathes in there is rather a harsh bark. It's not usually associated with a paroxysmal cough or vomiting, and it usually gets better in a few days.

My granddaughter has a bad cough that sounds very much like a whoop, and she sometimes vomits at the end of a coughing fit. Could this be whooping cough?

Yes. Although the phlegm in a bad cough can cause vomiting, it rarely causes a whoop. Take her to the doctor and keep her away from other children, particularly babies.

Is it possible to get whooping cough even after immunization?

Yes, but it's a much milder disease. It's more likely to recur in teenagers and adults who were immunized as babies, rather than in children.

My child has had convulsions, so the doctor won't give him whooping cough vaccine. Should my son also not have had the tetanus and diphtheria vaccine?

No. There is no evidence at all that the tetanus and diphtheria vaccine causes any neurological problems, and it is very important that he should have these and the polio vaccine that is usually given at the same time.

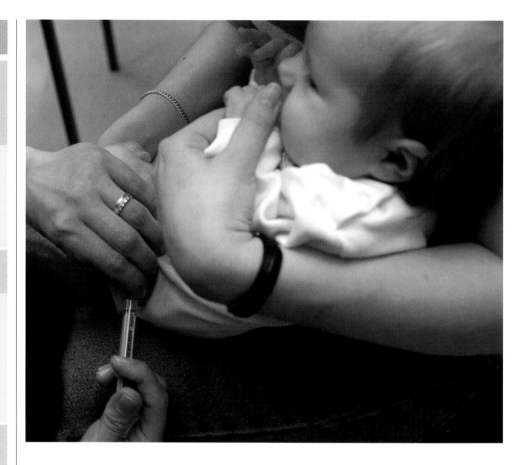

▲ *Whooping cough vaccine is most often given as part of a triple vaccine, the other two being diphtheria and tetanus, that is injected using a hypodermic syringe.*

drinks and meals; and no rushing about. Children who go blue during coughing bouts, or who cannot keep fluid down, need hospital admission for oxygen therapy, suction to remove mucus plugs, and replacement of fluids either by a tube through the nose into the stomach, or by injection into a vein (see Intravenous Infusion; Oxygen Therapy). Some doctors give a mild sedative to reduce coughing spells (see Sedatives).

Prevention

Lifelong prevention occurs only after an attack of whooping cough, so that pertussis can be prevented only by active immunization with the pertussis vaccine. The vaccine consists of a suspension of killed organisms of *Bordetella pertussis*. They stimulate the body to produce antibodies without actually giving rise to an attack of whooping cough.

The vaccine has to be given in three doses to give about 95 percent protection against the disease. The vaccine is more conveniently given at the same time as diphtheria and tetanus vaccine (hence the triple vaccine of diphtheria, tetanus, and pertussis—DPT or DPaT—given to most infants). According to the National Center for Health Statistics, in 2001, 82 percent of children between the ages of 19 months and 35 months received the DPT vaccination.

The American Academy of Pediatrics recommends that a course of five whooping cough vaccinations be given to children at four months, six months, 12 months, 15 to 18 months, and four to six years. Immunity from whooping cough wanes steadily after immunization and an additional booster dose is necessary for adolescents (15 to 17 years of age) and young adults (25 to 30 years of age). The purpose of these additional doses is to get rid of a reservoir of *Bordetella* organisms in older people, which is known to be a source of infection for young children.

The immunization controversy

Whooping cough was once common in the United States, but following the introduction of a vaccine in the 1940s and subsequent widespread immunization, its incidence declined. Since 1980, however, the incidence has been rising and there have been sporadic epidemics from time to time

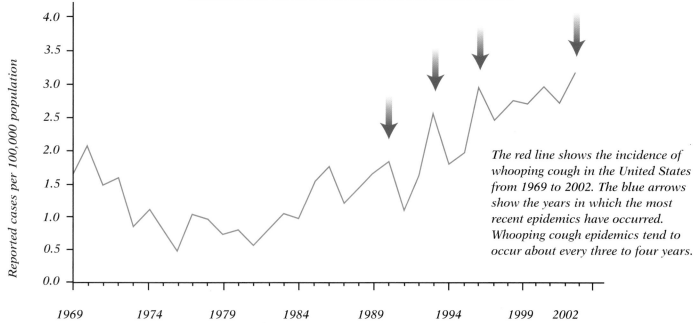

INCIDENCE OF WHOOPING COUGH IN THE UNITED STATES

The red line shows the incidence of whooping cough in the United States from 1969 to 2002. The blue arrows show the years in which the most recent epidemics have occurred. Whooping cough epidemics tend to occur about every three to four years.

as a result of failure of immunization programs, usually because of the fear of side effects. Also, the incidence of whooping cough among adolescents and adults has increased substantially because immunity diminishes in many adolescents and adults and no vaccine has been developed for these age groups. However, the death rate from whooping cough has been reduced by immunization to very low figures. Before a vaccine was available, whooping cough killed 5,000 to 10,000 people in the United States each year. Now the annual number of deaths is less than 20.

In view of these facts it is no longer acceptable that parents should be influenced by out-of-date information about the risks of immunization. In the mid-1970s, when vaccination against whooping cough had been widely used for about 16 years, reports began to appear about cases in which children had suffered convulsions and permanent brain damage attributed to such immunization. Because the same effects are a feature of the disease, there was no clear evidence that these cases were due to the immunization. However, severe anxiety among parents led to a widespread rejection of whooping cough immunization. The result was major whooping cough epidemics with the deaths of many young children.

Risks of immunization

The common adverse reactions from whooping cough vaccination consist mainly of swelling and redness at the site of the injection. A small, painless lump may form. This is of no consequence and will disappear in due course. Occasionally, the reaction takes the form of crying, screaming, and fever. Very occasionally, a child will become pale for a time and go limp. Convulsions sometimes occur, but these are not uncommon in children in the first year of life, whether they have been immunized or not.

In one major research study in Britain, the conclusion was that the number of cases was too small to provide conclusive evidence that the vaccine could cause permanent brain damage. Studies in the United States produced similar findings. In one of these a group of children who had seizures or floppy episodes within 38 hours of

vaccination were checked six or seven years later. None of them showed serious brain damage or intellectual impairment.

When not to vaccinate

Because of the risk of complications, pertussis vaccine should not be given to any child who has a fever or feverish illness (see Temperature); who has had convulsions, or whose parents or siblings have had convulsions; who has late development; or who has a known disorder of the central nervous system (see Nervous System). If there is any severe local or general reaction such as a very high temperature, confusion, odd behavior, or a convulsion after the first immunization, pertussis vaccine should be left out of subsequent vaccinations.

DPT and DPaT vaccines

Immunization against whooping cough is usually given in a combined form with a triple vaccine, known as DPT, that also protects against diphtheria and tetanus. Immunization in children is highly effective. Traditionally, the whooping cough vaccine has contained the *Bordetella* organism that has been killed by heat so that it cannot cause the disease. This is called whole cell vaccine, and it fairly often causes minor to moderate local reactions. A few unusually sensitive individuals have had seizures.

Because of concerns over these side effects, other whooping cough vaccines have been developed since the late 1970s and early 1980s. These contain purified extracts of the *Bordetella* organism and thus are called acellular vaccines. Several of these have been licensed for use in the United States. When combined with diphtheria and tetanus toxoids they are called DPaT vaccines. This is now the preferred form.

Acellular whooping cough vaccines are recommended for all children from four months onward. For most children of 15 months or more, however, the older DPT is an acceptable alternative.

See also: **Coughing; Fevers; Immunization; Incubation; Lung and lung diseases; Quarantine; Vaccinations**

Withdrawal symptoms

I've heard that people can become habituated rather than addicted to certain drugs. Will they have the same withdrawal symptoms once they quit the drug?

When a doctor refers to drugs to which patients can become habituated, he or she probably means those drugs that are habit-forming, including mild painkillers and laxatives. With addictive drugs, patients get severe withdrawal symptoms. However, when a patient comes off a habit-forming drug, he or she may have only a vague sense of unease and loss. Nevertheless, it can be almost as difficult to persuade someone to stop using a habit-forming drug as it is to persuade someone to stop a true addiction.

Why do some people go back on drugs once they've quit, especially after suffering such terrible withdrawal symptoms?

There are probably two main reasons for this. In the case of heroin withdrawal, there is a phase during which the acute withdrawal symptoms are over but there are still bodily changes resulting from long-term use of the drug. Breath control is not quite normal, and there may be such symptoms as premature orgasm or ejaculation. This phase may go on for some time, and addicts who are very distressed may seek immediate relief of these low-level symptoms by taking some of the drug. Second, the drug and the habit were once the central part of the addict's life, so if this keystone is removed, then something else must be put in its place. Otherwise, the social and psychological pressures that helped to foster the addiction will push the addict back to his or her old habit. The success of some community projects in getting people off drugs may be explained by their ability to replace the drug with something more meaningful in the addict's life.

Most people have seen vivid portrayals of the agonies of withdrawal from drugs or alcohol depicted in television programs and movies. Yet what actually happens during withdrawal, and what are the dangers to the addict?

Addictive drugs, however undesirable they may be, are deeply embedded in modern culture. Addictive drugs include not only so-called hard substances like heroin, morphine, and cocaine and crack (see Cocaine and Crack; Morphine), but also such everyday and socially acceptable drugs as alcohol and cigarettes. Once the addict attempts to end the addiction, he or she will suffer from withdrawal symptoms. Most of these symptoms can be very unpleasant and, in rare cases, even fatal. Above all, the addict will have to have great strength of character, combined with medical treatment, to be able to survive the withdrawal from the addictive drug.

What is addiction?

Drug addiction has a number of characteristics. When there is true physical dependence, an addict will experience a physical illness that can be recognized as withdrawal when the drug is stopped. Further, addicts will develop what is known as tolerance to their addictive drug. This means that they gradually end up taking huge amounts without suffering from the effects that could quite possibly kill a nonaddict.

One peculiar aspect of addiction serves to underline how it may be regarded as a state of mind in the drug user. Most addicts admit that they found the first experience of their drug rather unpleasant. This is particularly so with morphine and heroin, but it is also true of cigarettes: few smokers can honestly say they enjoyed their first cigarette. Something in the addict's state of mind or social circumstances causes the addict to persist with a habit despite the side effects and until need for the drug is built up (see Side Effects).

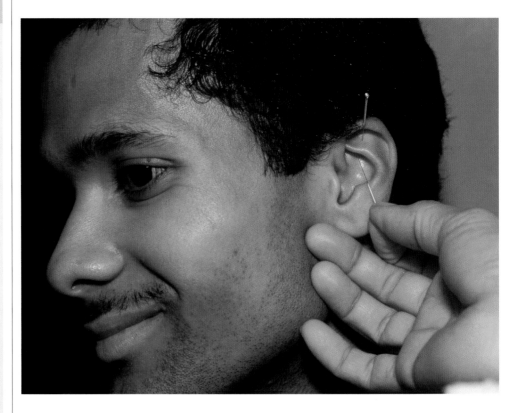

▲ *Acupuncture needles are being inserted into the ear of a drug addict as a form of treatment in a drug rehabilitation program at the Lincoln Hospital in Bronx, New York.*

Morphine and heroin

There are two separate aspects to the withdrawal of these drugs. First, the patient will go to extreme lengths to try to get a further dose of the drug, while the level of his or her anxiety will increase as the time for a fix approaches (see Anxiety). Second, the addict will experience very specific physical symptoms once the drug is withdrawn. These include tears, a runny nose, and sweating (occurring about eight hours after the last dose), followed by a period of restlessness and disturbed sleep. Upon waking, the addict will have more severe symptoms such as uncontrollable trembling, goose bumps, and irritability that can often result in violent behavior.

The real crisis time occurs after about 48 hours. The addict will suffer a runny nose as during a bad cold, sweating, goose bumps, muscle spasms that cause sudden and uncontrollable kicking, excessive yawning, abdominal pains (see Abdomen), and diarrhea. The addict is extremely weak and depressed at this stage, but there may be uncontrolled activity of the nervous system, with ejaculation in men and orgasm in women (see Erection and Ejaculation; Nervous System; Orgasm). Occasionally, the blood pressure falls sharply, causing collapse and sometimes even death (see Blood Pressure).

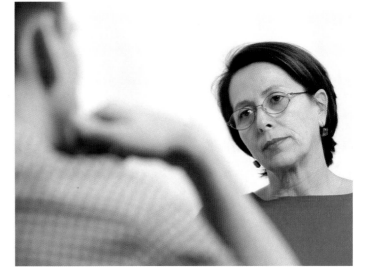

▲ *Before giving up a drug, a patient should consult a doctor to find out what sort of withdrawal symptoms can be expected.*

Withdrawal symptoms

DRUG	SYMPTOMS	DURATION OF SYMPTOMS	TREATMENT
Morphine and related drugs such as heroin	Symptoms start at the time that the next dose is due and include increasing anxiety. Other symptoms include sweating, goose bumps, trembling, and disturbed sleep. Later, muscle spasms, abdominal pains, and diarrhea may set in.	Symptoms last for a varying length of time depending on the duration of action of the drug. With heroin, the symptoms start after a few hours and they are at their height between 36 and 72 hours later. This is followed by a period which may last for weeks or months when there may be disturbances of bodily functions.	Symptoms can be stopped at any time with a dose of an opiate drug. Many treatment centers like to change from heroin to methadone before withdrawal is attempted.
Barbiturates	Restlessness, anxiety, trembling, confusion, vomiting, and disturbed sleep. Convulsions often occur. Roughly half of patients go on to develop a full-blown delirium.	Duration depends on which drug is used: symptoms last longer in long-acting drugs. If delirium occurs, it is usually on the third day. Four or five days may be required for full recovery.	The addictive drug will stop the attack at any time; therefore, a gradual lowering of the dose is used. Once the delirium occurs, no drug is able to stop it.
Alcohol	Mild: trembling relieved by another drink. Moderate: anxiety and hallucinations. Severe: fits and delirium tremens (DTs) with severe hallucinations. Collapse and death are not uncommon.	Minor withdrawal shaking can be seen after a drinking bout and resolves within a few hours. Moderate symptoms take a day or so to get better, but DTs may take up to a week.	Like other drugs, alcohol itself will stop the symptoms. Minor symptoms can be relieved with a drug called chlormethiazole: this has replaced the practice of giving small doses of alcohol during withdrawal. DTs must be allowed to run their course.
Cocaine and crack	Irritability and tiredness. Long-term users can suffer from depression.	Uncertain. Depression can be long-lasting.	None
Amphetamines and other stimulants	Sleepiness, lassitude, overeating, agitation, and depression	Similar to cocaine and crack	None
Tobacco	Irritability, anxiety, and overeating	May last for weeks	Nicotine chewing gum may help people get over the withdrawal symptoms

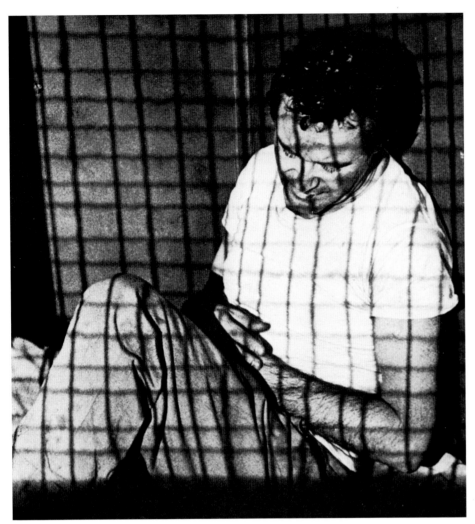

▲ *Withdrawal symptoms from alcohol, as seen in this still from the movie* **The Days of Wine and Roses,** *can be similar to those of heroin.*

On the third day, the patient may have full-blown delirium tremens (DTs). During this time the patient is delirious and often hyperthermic (overheated). As with heroin withdrawal, collapse of the circulation can occur, which can be fatal. Fits often result from the withdrawal of alcohol and are almost inevitable if barbiturates are suddenly stopped (see Convulsions).

Crack and cocaine

Occasional users of cocaine suffer few and minor withdrawal symptoms. These commonly amount to no more than a degree of irritability and lassitude and a desire to indulge again in the drug. Long-term users may suffer more marked withdrawal effects. There may be severe depression. The withdrawal effects of cocaine are virtually the same as those of amphetamine (see box on page 2417; see also Amphetamines).

Treatment

During withdrawal from morphine and heroin, symptoms are made less unpleasant by giving the addict a morphinelike drug called methadone, which is taken by mouth. Because this drug persists longer in the body, the symptoms do not come on so suddenly or so severely, although they will actually last longer. Gradual reduction of the dose over weeks or months also helps reduce the severity of the symptoms.

In alcohol withdrawal, a drug called chlormethiazole may help to reduce or even abolish the symptoms. The drug can also be used in barbiturate withdrawal. However, it is unable to stop DTs once they have developed.

The symptoms recede after a week or 10 days. After this, though, it is still possible to detect the effect of the drug on the body: for example, breath control is disturbed (see Breathing), and there is an exaggerated increase in breathing as the amount of carbon dioxide in the blood rises. The addict is very likely to go back to drugs during this second phase. In fact, this vulnerability represents continuing bodily dependence on the drug, and it is during this phase that the addict trying to break the habit needs most support.

Alcohol and barbiturates

The symptoms of barbiturate withdrawal are very similar to those of alcohol withdrawal. The first stage of alcohol withdrawal may occur in people who drink only moderately, but who have had one or two heavy drinking sessions in the course of the previous few days. There is often a pronounced shaking of the hands, which is relieved by taking another drink. This alcoholic tremor is a definite sign that drinking is getting beyond control and should be stopped or, at the very least, cut down.

The next stage is one of anxiety and agitation. This occurs only in chronically heavy drinkers and happens about 24 hours after the last drink. The addict may begin to have hallucinations, which can be very frightening.

Perhaps the most common withdrawal symptoms occur on quitting smoking. These include irritability and anxiety, and a tendency to eat more and put on weight. Smokers can be helped by nicotine chewing gum. Nicotine seems to be one of the main addictive factors, although it is only one of about 3,000 compounds in cigarette smoke. Once smokers have stopped cigarettes and changed over to the gum, they may find it easy to go on reducing the amount of gum until they are using none at all (see Smoking).

In cases of addiction to drugs, alcohol, or barbiturates, however, even after withdrawal symptoms have abated, there is often a need to continue treatment, usually in the form of rehabilitation. Willpower on its own may not be enough, especially if addiction has involved a hard drug such as morphine or heroin (see Rehabilitation).

Most developed countries have social machinery to combat both drug addiction and alcoholic problems, and a backup program that provides reinforcement and support is a vital addition to this.

See also: **Alcoholism; Barbiturates; Drug abuse; Hallucinations; Heroin; Nicotine**

Worms

Throughout the world worms constitute a major health problem. Although few serious types of infestation are likely to occur in temperate climates, in the tropics worms cause a wide range of debilitating diseases.

Hygiene is important, since many roundworms are spread by food or water contaminated with human feces. Hookworm can be avoided by wearing shoes. Many filarial worms are spread by bloodsucking insects, so try to avoid insect bites.

Yes, some worms can be avoided by cooking food thoroughly. Both the common tapeworms are spread by undercooked beef and pork. The larvae die at 144°F (62°C), so very high temperatures are not necessary. A tapeworm found in fish (*Diphyllobothrium latum*) occurs in Scandinavia; it is caught by eating raw fish. *Anisakis marina* is a parasite of herrings that can be ingested with raw fish; it infects humans in Holland and Japan, where raw herring and sushi are eaten. There are also two forms of liver fluke in Asia that can be caught only by eating raw or undercooked fish.

Although roundworms are most common in the tropics, the United States has up to four million cases of ascariasis each year. Drugs are used to kill the roundworms in the intestines.

Common among young children, pinworms live in the intestines, and eggs are deposited near the anus. Severe anal itching occurs; the eggs are transmitted from the fingernails to bedding, clothing, food, or the air. Treatment is by two doses of piperazine, and usually involves the entire family.

Worms are referred to as helminths. They are multicelled animals as opposed to single-celled bacteria (see Bacteria) and protozoa that are the other main parasites (see Parasites) of humans. Of the parasitic worms, most species have a specific life cycle that allows infestation to continue and to pass through another animal before infesting a human host. For example, schistosomes, which cause schistosomiasis, pass through a phase of development in a water snail before infesting humans.

Some of the worms that cause trouble in humans use another animal as their primary host. The host is the animal in which the worm reaches its adult form, and any animal that it infects during the egg or larval stage is called the intermediate host. In this way, the larvae of the echinococcus worm, which infests dogs, may be passed in the larval stage to humans, forming a hydatid cyst that develops in the human liver.

Helminths that cause problems in humans are divided into three major groups. The first of these are the nematodes or roundworms that cause such diseases as elephantiasis. Second are the cestodes or tapeworms; and third, the trematodes, or flatworms, which give rise to schistosomiasis and liver fluke infestation. The cestodes and trematodes have similar life cycles.

Nematodes

The nematodes have a wide range of shapes and sizes and great variability in the way their life cycles work. Those of medical importance to humans include various types of roundworm.

Filariae are a very important group of worms that cause such diseases as elephantiasis (see Elephantiasis) and river blindness. The adult worms are round, and both males and females need to be present in the primary host so that reproduction can take place. These worms are carried from person to person by a bloodsucking insect, with a different insect species for each species of worm.

In general, the pattern is that the adult worms mate and the female produces a large number of larvae, or microfilariae, which swarm into the human host's bloodstream. If an insect bites the infected human, microfilariae are taken in with the blood. These develop in the mosquito, and are injected back into another human, setting up a new infestation and spreading the infection.

Hookworms are very common throughout the tropics and subtropics. The different forms have a similar life cycle, in which an adult worm lives in the duodenum (part of the small intestine) where it feeds on blood and lays its eggs. These then pass out in feces. In warm soil the eggs change into larvae, which can penetrate human skin when bare feet come in contact with it.

Once in the bloodstream, the larvae are carried to the lungs. They then travel up the windpipe to be swallowed and find their way to the intestine. There is often severe itching (see Itches) at the entry point. Hookworm

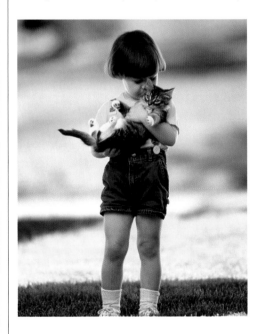

▲ *Young children are at risk of picking up roundworm larvae from cats and dogs. Parents should ensure that strict rules of hygiene are applied to both children and pets.*

► *A number of roundworms live in human intestines at some stage in their life cycle. They include the ascaris adult (bottom right) and larva (inset), whipworms (far right), and the hookworm (right), whose larva penetrates the skin.*

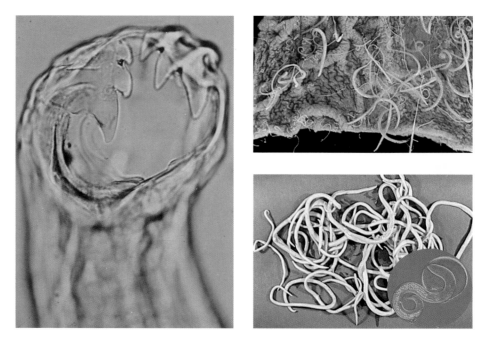

larvae of other species, such as the dog hookworm, may find their way through the skin and at the point of entry cause a rash called a larva migrans (see Rashes).

Ascaris cause a large number of infestations, and it has been estimated that up to one-quarter of the world's population may be infected with ascaris. The eggs are ingested directly from food that is contaminated with feces (see Feces). The worms live in the intestine. Once a larva hatches in the duodenum, it gets into the bloodstream and imbeds itself in the lungs. From here it is coughed up the windpipe and swallowed. Ascaris causes few symptoms in most people, but there may be inflammation of the lungs as the larvae pass through. Large numbers of ascaris in the intestine can certainly cause abdominal symptoms and lead to blockage of the intestine.

Pinworms, common all over the world, also live in the intestines. The adult female worm emerges from the anus to lay eggs that then cause irritation. The infested person has probably picked up the eggs on the fingers when scratching and inadvertently swallowed them. This may lead to reinfection of the same person and to infection of others, which is a situation most common in children. The main symptom that the patient notices is anal itching.

HOW WORMS INFEST HUMANS

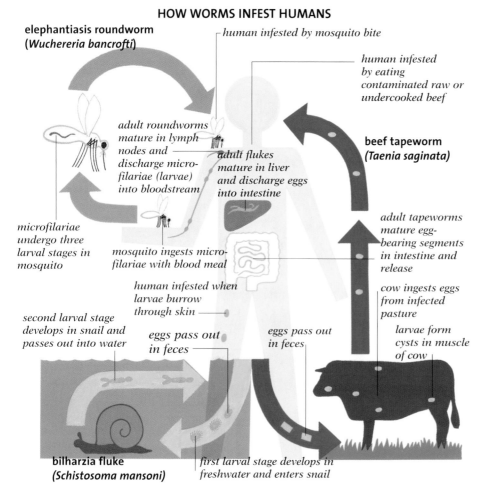

elephantiasis roundworm (*Wuchereria bancrofti*)

human infested by mosquito bite

human infested by eating contaminated raw or undercooked beef

adult roundworms mature in lymph nodes and discharge micro-filariae (larvae) into bloodstream

adult flukes mature in liver and discharge eggs into intestine

beef tapeworm (*Taenia saginata*)

microfilariae undergo three larval stages in mosquito

adult tapeworms mature egg-bearing segments in intestine and release

mosquito ingests micro-filariae with blood meal

human infested when larvae burrow through skin

cow ingests eggs from infected pasture

second larval stage develops in snail and passes out into water

eggs pass out in feces

eggs pass out in feces

larvae form cysts in muscle of cow

bilharzia fluke (*Schistosoma mansoni*)

first larval stage develops in freshwater and enters snail

Trematodes (flatworms or flukes)

Bilharzia (schistosomiasis) is one of the diseases caused by a trematode. The Egyptian form affects the bladder (see Bladder and Bladder Problems) because the bladder is where the eggs of the organism cause inflammation when they hatch into adult worms.

Another two forms of the disease infest the large intestine. Eggs are passed out in the feces and develop in water snails before the larvae find their way back into the human body by burrowing into the skin. The liver fluke is another trematode (see Liver Fluke) that causes problems, especially in Southeast Asia where raw fish (called sushi in Japan) is a popular delicacy.

Cestodes (tapeworms)

Tapeworms affect only meat-eaters. The typical tapeworm is the beef tapeworm, *Taenia saginata*. Humans are the primary host, and the worm anchors itself to the wall

◄ *Transmission of worms to humans occurs in three ways: from an insect carrier, such as a mosquito; from the infested meat or feces of an animal; or directly via the skin, as in the case of the bilharzia fluke.*

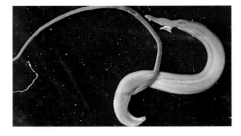

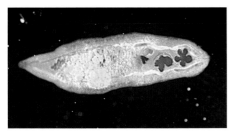

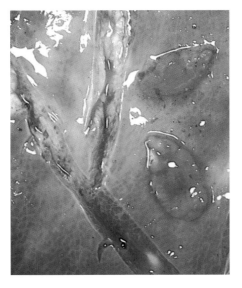

◄ The bilharzia fluke (top far left) lays its eggs in the human intestine, but humans are only rarely hosts of liver flukes, which are carried by other animals. Fasciola hepatica *(left) infests cattle;* Opisthrocus viverina *(bottom far left) lives in fish.*

Treatment and control

Drugs are available to kill most worms that infect humans, but some of the drugs used are toxic. Worm infestation is a major public health problem, but control rather than cure is the answer. Many sorts of infestation could be avoided by better sanitation (see Infection and Infectious Diseases) and by reducing the risk of food and water being contaminated with human feces. In other cases controlling the intermediate host would cut down the risk of disease. For example, the Chinese have made great strides in reducing the risk of getting schistosomiasis by vastly reducing the population of water snails.

of the upper intestine, producing a long string of egg-bearing segments (the tape). Eggs pass out in the feces, and for the infestation to be passed on they must be eaten by some suitable intermediate host such as a cow. In the intermediate host they hatch into larvae, which spread to invade all the muscles. The life cycle continues if a human eats the infested uncooked flesh.

Despite the enormous size they may reach, sometimes up to 30 feet (9 m), tapeworms produce few symptoms. The eggs of the pig tapeworm, *Taenia solium*, may, however, pass into the bloodstream.

See also: **Public health**

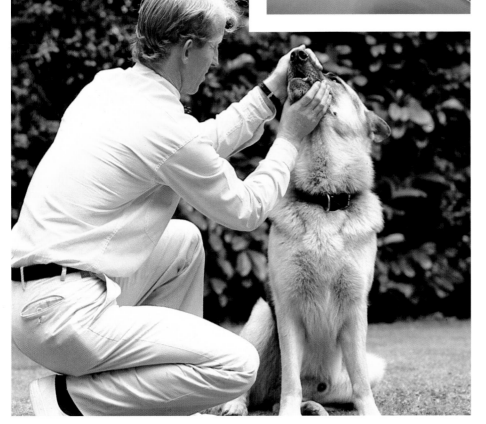

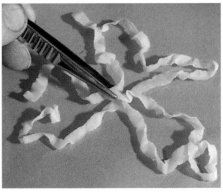

◄▼ The dog tapeworm (left) can be transmitted to humans; prevention lies in worming all dogs regularly (bottom left). In most cases, however, human tapeworms (below) are the result of eating partly cooked or raw meat and fish. The eggs of Taenia solium *(bottom), a pig tapeworm, can cause the serious disease cysticerosis.*

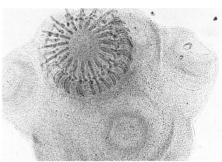

Wounds

I bruise very easily. Is there anything that I can do about this?

Some people do bruise more easily than others, probably because the capillaries in the skin are more fragile. Most people who bruise easily are perfectly healthy, and the condition is just a nuisance that has to be lived with. Only in rare cases is bruising a sign of blood clotting disorders or vitamin deficiency.

How does one control bleeding?

Apply pressure directly onto the bleeding area. This stops the bleeding and allows clotting of blood in the wound within a few minutes. In a leg or an arm wound it is also helpful to elevate the part as high as possible (this reduces the blood pressure in the limb). Tourniquets should be avoided, since they can do great damage if applied by someone inexperienced.

When I had a deep cut, the doctor sutured it with dissolving stitches. How do these work?

Dissolving stitches are strong when they are put in, but gradually begin to soften up in the body. As they dissolve, the body's cells remove the small pieces of debris, and the stitch eventually disappears. Dissolving stitches are often used inside the body; they tend to make slightly more scar tissue, so they are not usually used on the parts of skin where a fine scar is preferable.

Do only deep cuts create scars?

Yes. A cut has to go through all the layers of skin to cause scarring. The outer layer of skin (epidermis) is largely made up of dead cells that come up from the deeper layer of the skin. If only the outer layer is damaged, as in a shallow cut or graze, the damage is repaired by cells moving up from the dermis, and no scarring occurs.

The seriousness of a wound depends on what part of the body it affects rather than its actual size. A small puncture to a vital organ like the heart or brain may cause death, whereas a large wound on the skin may have no lasting effects.

Wounds fall into several categories: abrasions, contusions, lacerations, incisions, and punctures. Gunshot wounds can have one or more features of these, but are included here because they very often require specialist treatment.

Abrasion: An abrasion is a graze. It occurs when the skin is rubbed forcibly against something rough. The outer layer of the skin, or epidermis, is rubbed away, exposing the deeper layer, or dermis. This deeper layer contains small blood vessels (capillaries), so a little bleeding occurs (see Capillaries). It also contains many nerve endings and these are left exposed by the graze, resulting in the intense stinging pain that accompanies such wounds.

Contusion: A contusion is a bruise. It occurs when a part of the body is struck by something blunt, leaving the skin unbroken. The tissues beneath the skin—the fat, muscles, and internal organs—receive the force of the blow. Small blood vessels in these tissues burst, and blood leaks into the tissues, causing them to swell and become tight. When this happens, further bleeding stops, but the tightening tissue causes pain. The blood that seeps into the tissues gradually loses most of the oxygen that it is carrying and, as it does so, turns a bluish-black color. This is why bruises are dark blue to black at first. Later the blood is broken down and reabsorbed by the body, and the bruise gradually becomes greenish-yellow or light yellow. Occasionally, the blood collects in a pool among the tissues rather than weeping out into the tissues. This is called a hematoma.

Gunshot wounds: These, and wounds caused by bomb blast shrapnel, cause extensive damage to tissue, and are particularly likely to become infected. The amount of damage a bullet causes obviously depends on the type of tissues through which the bullet passes. The speed of the bullet is important. Low-velocity bullets (for example, those fired by handguns) tend to damage only those tissues through which the bullet actually passes. High-velocity bullets (most rifle bullets, for example) create a shock wave as they pass, and can cause serious damage to tissues lying at some distance from the bullet track itself.

Laceration: A laceration means a tear, but it is commonly used to refer to any sort of cut. Lacerations can vary from a trivial wound that just goes through the skin to very deep wounds involving such important structures as tendons, blood vessels, and nerves (see Tendons). Lacerations can occur through contact with something sharp, such as a knife or a piece of glass;

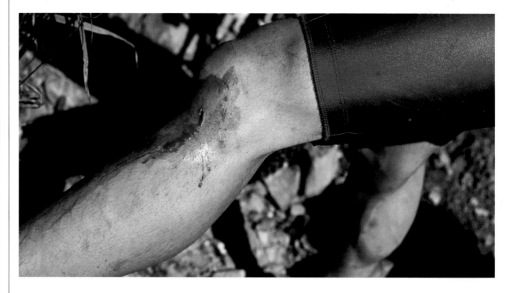

▲ *This wound, received from mountain biking, is both a laceration and an abrasion.*

or they can occur with a blunt blow: for example, striking the forehead on the floor may split open the skin.

Incision: This word is commonly used to mean a cut made with a clean sharp instrument as in surgery. Therefore, the only difference between an incision and a laceration is that an incision is intentional, as in a surgical operation, and the damage is limited to those actual tissues that were intended to be cut.

Puncture: A puncture is a wound made by a pointed object such as a needle or a thorn. Punctures are deeper than they are wide, and serious damage can be done to deep structures without much obvious damage on the surface. Because these wounds are often made by long, thin objects, it is common for a little piece of the object to break off inside, leaving a foreign body.

Wound healing

Wounds heal in one of two ways: either they resolve completely, leaving no trace, or they heal by scarring.

A wound can heal without leaving a trace only if the wounded tissue has not been entirely disrupted. Grazes heal in this way because only the top layer of the skin is rubbed away, leaving intact the deeper layer. This deeper layer contains the cells that multiply to form the top layer, and when the top layer has been damaged this process continues until normal skin has been restored. Occasionally, the site of a deep graze is visible years later as a slightly pale area of skin.

Contusions also heal completely, since the wound consists mainly of blood seeping into the tissues. This blood is broken down and absorbed by the body, so bruises gradually soften and disappear. Since the structures in the bruised area are not damaged, no scarring results.

Other types of wound heal by scarring. When the injury occurs, there is a gap in the tissue that becomes filled with blood. This blood becomes clotted and, soon after, the blood clot is invaded by cells called fibroblasts. These cells produce a simple type of fibrous tissue that helps to tie the sides of the wound together. At the same time, the fibrous tissue is penetrated by small blood vessels from the

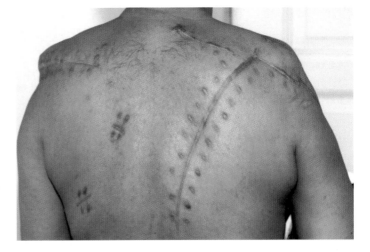

▲ *The Indonesian journalist Abi Kusno Nachran got these scars from lacerations received by a machete in revenge for his reports on the illegal timber trade. He had to have 209 stitches.*

surrounding tissues. This blood supply brings with it more fiber-producing cells, as well as a good supply of raw materials: oxygen, protein, sugar, and so on. The healing wound is a very busy area at this early stage of healing, and this is shown by the fact that a healing wound is slightly swollen and firm, and the scar is bright red to pink. Over the next few months the early fibrous tissue becomes more highly organized, with the protein fibers lined up to resist the stresses in the wound, and the scar becomes softer and whiter. In some areas, scars become almost invisible and blend in well with the surrounding tissue (a good example is a scar on the palm of the hand). In other areas, such as the abdomen and chest, the scar tends to widen as it heals, leaving a permanent, obvious scar.

In relatively simple tissues such as skin or fat, a small scar has little or no effect, but in more specialized tissues, scarring may stop their function altogether. For example, if a nerve is cut then stitched back together, impulses passing along it from the brain can still flow, but if the area fills with scar tissue the nerve will not work. Special techniques for repairing nerves can minimize this problem.

▼ *Bullfighting is deliberately undertaken for its danger: the matador runs the risk of being gored (punctured and lacerated) by the bull's horns, or even killed, every time he enters the ring.*

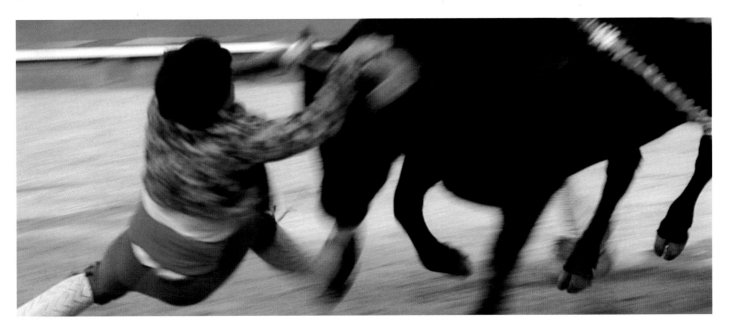

Questions and Answers

I bruised my hip very badly in a fall and now it is very painful. Is it possible that I have broken my hip?

Yes. Bruising is a feature of broken bones because the bone actually bleeds into the surrounding tissues. This shows on the surface as bruising. If the break in the bone has not actually come apart it is possible to use the limb, although it will continue to be painful until the fracture heals. The danger is that the fracture may come apart, so it would be best to see your doctor.

I stepped on a nail in the yard. Should I have a tetanus injection?

Tetanus is a very serious type of infection caused by bacteria that live in soil and animal excrement. The infection can be prevented by a vaccine that is usually given in childhood. It is necessary to have a booster shot every 10 years to keep up your resistance, so if you have not had a booster it would be wise to have it now.

Why does an eye turn black when it is injured?

A black eye is really a bruise. When bruising occurs, blood leaks out of the small blood vessels in the injured area. This blood rapidly gives off the oxygen it is carrying, and as it does so it changes from bright red to dark blue-black. It is this color that shows through the skin as a bruise. The tissues around the eye are very loose and the overlying skin is thin, so a black eye swells up dramatically and may become very dark in color.

When I grazed my arm recently my mother said I should not cover the wound. Was she right?

Yes. It is usually best to allow a graze to dry up. Over the first few hours it will form a dry scab that serves as a very effective dressing. Covering a graze makes the area moist, favoring the development of infection.

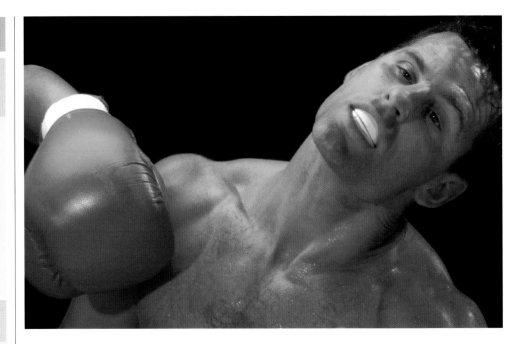

▲ *Sports injuries are common and take a variety of forms. A blow to the face, for example, causes bruises and swelling, so a cold compress is a soothing remedy.*

Treatment

Nature is a great healer of wounds. Any treatment given does not affect this healing process, but it sets the stage for healing without complications, and with a minimum of side effects.

Abrasions: These generally heal quickly and completely. The only treatment that is required is cleansing of the wound followed, in some cases, by a dressing. Cleansing can be done with a mild soap and water (cold water is more soothing). Ideally, the graze should then be left exposed to the air. Within a few hours a tough scab forms over it, acting as a natural protective dressing. However, in some cases it may be better to cover the graze with a dressing to prevent it from rubbing on clothes or becoming dirty. Plastic materials tend to keep the graze moist and dark, favoring infection, so a porous material is better.

Contusions: These require little attention. A cold compress or ice pack applied as soon as possible after the injury helps prevent swelling. This is particularly effective, for example, in a black eye (see Black Eye; Swellings). Bruises heal eventually and not much can be done to hasten this process.

▼ *This abdominal scar is the result of a spear wound on a native Brazilian patient that turned septic. Medical treatment was needed to clean the wound so it could heal.*

▼ *A bad fracture can cause a serious external wound. This leg was operated on, and antibiotic beads were placed in the wound to combat infection before suturing.*

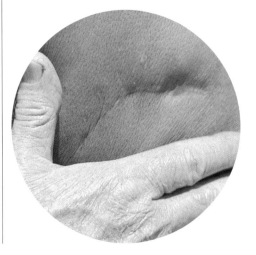

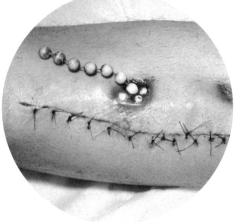

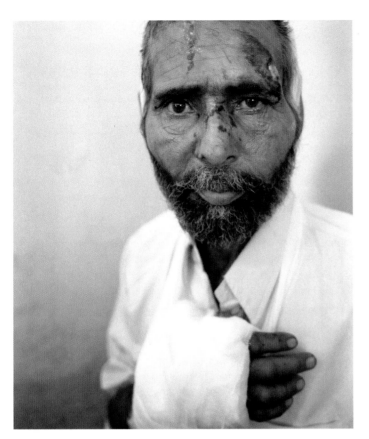

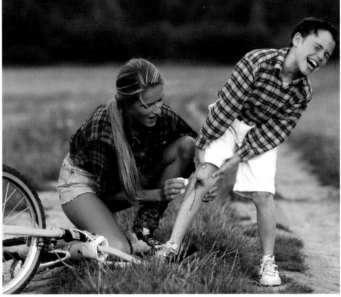

▲ *This mother is wise to try to clean her son's wound as soon as possible after his fall from a bicycle.*

◄ *This man has received a number of wounds, but a dressing has been put on those wounds that are most likely to come into contact with dirt and to rub against clothing.*

Gunshot wounds: Treatment consists of early surgery to explore the path of the bullet. All tissue that has been so badly damaged that it cannot survive must be removed at this first operation. It is often necessary to remove large amounts of tissue, or even to amputate a limb, in order to achieve a clean wound. Major bleeding must be stopped, and damaged vessels repaired to ensure a blood supply to the surrounding tissues. Damaged intestine must be removed to prevent leakage and serious infection, and broken bones must be cleansed, splinted, or put in traction (see Splints; Traction). Complicated surgery to reconstruct damaged tissue is left to a later date. Initial surgery is performed to save life and to set the stage for a clean, healthy wound. Techniques for treating major gunshot wounds have improved greatly in recent years, so that most people who reach the hospital alive now survive and recover.

Lacerations: These often need treatment. Bleeding is best controlled by direct pressure over the cut, using clean gauze or cloth. Elevation of the lacerated part helps reduce bleeding. Firm pressure applied for several minutes generally stops bleeding from small vessels. If a larger vessel is cut, continuous pressure may be necessary until the victim reaches the hospital. Even if a large artery is cut, it is better to apply the pressure directly to the wound rather than to use a tourniquet. This is because a tourniquet can do serious damage both in the tissues that are being squeezed and in the rest of the limb that is having its blood supply stopped.

Because all tissues have a certain degree of elasticity, any cut tends to retract or become larger. For example, a straight cut of 6 inches (15 cm) to the skin becomes a wound 6 inches by 1 inch (15 cm by 2.5 cm) wide. This is why many lacerations need to be stitched together to allow the cut edges to heal in the shortest time and with the smallest possible scar. The stitches need to be left in place for a long enough time for healing to make the wound strong enough to hold itself together. In a wound that has merely gone through the skin, only the skin itself is stitched. In deeper wounds, several layers of tissue may be divided, and each layer is stitched separately.

There are two principal types of stitches: that is, absorbable and nonabsorbable. Absorbable stitches are made from materials that dissolve slowly and that can be removed by the body, the most common being catgut, which is in fact made from sheep's intestines. Nonabsorbable sutures are made from silk, nylon, or steel. The type of suture that is used depends on the judgment of the doctor. As a general rule, nonabsorbable sutures are stronger and are less likely to react in the tissues, but absorbable sutures are convenient because they do not need to be removed.

Dressings for lacerations may be the only treatment needed, or they may be used after stitching. A firm dressing will help stop bleeding and make the wound more comfortable. Adhesive strips may be used instead of stitches to pull the wound together. In general, dressings are used as a protection against rubbing or knocking the wound while it is healing. There are many types of dressing materials, but none has any magical effect on wound healing. Often, leaving the wound open to the air is as good a treatment as any.

Puncture: A puncture wound needs treatment if the puncturing object is large or dirty. Because the wound is deep, it is easy to underestimate the amount of damage by looking only at the surface. It may be necessary for the track of the puncture to be opened by means of surgery and any damaged tissue cleansed and repaired.

Complications

Whenever the skin is broken, bacteria enter the wound from outside (see Bacteria). Whether these bacteria actually cause an infection depends on their strength and number, and on the ability of the tissues to resist the bacteria. Of these two factors, the most important is the resistance. For example, a young healthy person who gets a cut on a fingertip rarely gets an infection in the wound, since the tissues have a good blood supply and his or her defenses take care of any bacteria that get into the cut (see Infection and Infectious Diseases).

If a wound contains a lot of badly damaged tissue, infection is much more likely to occur. The damaged tissue will have a poor blood supply, so the body's cells may have difficulty in reaching the area where infection is beginning. The bacteria actually feed and multiply on the dead tissue, and as they multiply they will begin to break down and destroy previously normal tissue.

Symptoms of a wound infection take 24 to 48 hours to develop after the injury. The victim notices increasing pain in the wound as the infection causes swelling and tightness in the tissues. The pain becomes constant and throbbing, while the wound itself swells and becomes red and hot. Later, fluid may begin to escape from the wound. Initially, this is clear fluid, but later it may become pus. The victim will feel unwell and may have a fever.

The best treatment for an infected wound is prevention. Any wound should be thoroughly cleansed. Superficial wounds need only be washed with mild soap or an antiseptic. Deeper wounds should be examined by a doctor. If there is dirt ground into the tissues, or if there is a lot of bruised, crushed tissue, all this will need to be removed, leaving clean healthy tissue. If the wound is very dirty, antibiotics may be given (see Antibiotics).

In established wound infections, the wound must be opened up so that any fluid or pus can drain away, and the dead and damaged tissue can be removed. If the wound has previously been sutured, the stitches are generally removed. It may be helpful to elevate the infected area, since this helps to get rid of the swelling. Antibiotics should be taken until the wound has calmed down (a minimum of five days).

One particular type of infection that must be guarded against is lockjaw, or tetanus. The tetanus bacteria give off tiny spores that are

▼ *This man—who jumped from a burning apartment building that was hit by a plane in Santa Monica, California—will need to have his wounds cleaned and stitched to help avoid scarring.*

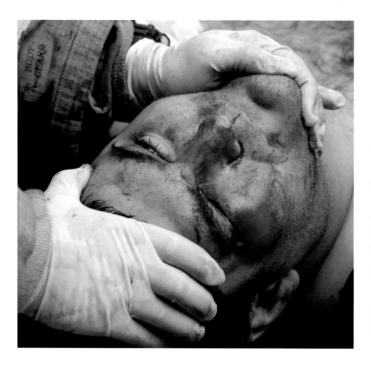

First aid in multiple injuries

Check breathing. Make sure the airways are clear: there may be false teeth, chewing gum, or blood blocking the throat. If breathing has stopped, begin mouth-to-mouth resuscitation.

If the victim is unconscious, roll him or her gently onto his or her side. This helps to keep the breathing tubes clear.

Control areas of bleeding by applying direct pressure on each wound. This may require several pairs of hands, each person concentrating on one wound.

Support any obvious fractures with splints, cushions, or blankets.

Seek expert medical help.

very hardy and live in soil and animal excrement. If the spores become established in a wound, they give off toxins that attack the nervous system, causing severe muscle spasms. Muscle spasm attacking the jaw muscles causes a forcible biting action, hence the term "lockjaw." Once this condition starts, treatment is difficult and many victims die. Lockjaw is prevented by cleaning wounds thoroughly and giving vaccine against tetanus (see Vaccinations). Most people receive the vaccine as children, and booster shots are needed every 10 years to maintain resistance. In practice, most people receive a booster only when they actually suffer a wound, rather than being vaccinated regularly.

Another complication is foreign bodies. This includes any piece of foreign material that is left behind in a wound. Foreign bodies cause two problems: they may press on important structures, causing pain and damage, and they cause inflammation in the tissues (see Inflammation). The cells of the body are able to recognize when a piece of foreign material is present, and then try to get rid of the intruding body. This process results in inflammation, which continues until the foreign body is removed. Some foreign material is inert: that is, it does not cause much of this type of reaction. Stainless steel and glass can remain in the body for years with little or no reaction. Biological materials such as cloth or wood cause very intense reactions, and must be removed for this reason.

It is a common belief that foreign bodies such as needles move around in the body, and may end up lodged in a vital organ. In fact, this does not happen. A needle or a piece of glass in the hand or foot (see Splinters) usually needs to be removed because it hurts when the person is standing or gripping, but the same foreign body in a large muscle such as the thigh is best left alone, since it will never cause any harm. Many war veterans have shrapnel embedded in various parts of their bodies for decades without suffering any ill effects. It is important to remove foreign bodies if infection is present, since they tend to maintain an infection despite treatment, therefore impeding wound healing.

See also: Abrasions and cuts; Bruises; Dressings and bandages; Healing; Lacerations; Scars; Skin and skin diseases; Surgery; Sutures; Tetanus

Wrinkles

Questions and Answers

Why do some people get wrinkles earlier than others?

Prolonged exposure to the sun is one of the causes of wrinkling. People who work outdoors tend to get wrinkles earlier than those who work indoors. Skin pigmentation gives protection; people with darker skins are less prone to wrinkling than fair-skinned people. Other factors that influence the early development of wrinkles are a poor diet, ill health, smoking, and poor skin care.

Will doing facial exercises delay the onset of wrinkles?

Almost certainly not. Some people believe that facial exercises stimulate muscle growth, tighten the skin, and prevent wrinkles. Others claim that the overuse of facial expressions accelerates wrinkling, since a pattern of facial lines will be fixed. In fact there are no muscles in the skin, so the effect of strengthening the facial muscles lying under the skin would be to stretch it a little.

Does skin cream containing collagen prevent wrinkles?

Collagen is a component of healthy skin, but wrinkling is believed to be caused by changes in skin structure. There is little scientific basis for the claim that collagen can rejuvenate skin. Creams with collagen may delay the appearance of wrinkles, but the effect may be due to the moisturizing properties of the cream rather than its collagen.

Can heavy bags under the eyes be surgically removed?

Yes. This operation is called a blepharoplasty and is like a face lift. Excess skin and fat are removed, and the remaining skin stretched and restitched.

Like graying hair, the appearance of a few wrinkles is a classic sign of aging. How do they come about, and can anything be done to avoid or put off this universal, and seemingly inevitable, phenomenon?

Skin wrinkling is usually apparent in anyone over 40, and often first occurs much earlier. Although wrinkles can give the face character, many people feel they are something to be avoided or postponed (see Skin and Skin Diseases).

Causes

The most important underlying change that brings about wrinkling involves the connective tissues just under the outer layer of the skin, which are made up of two types of protein fiber: collagen and elastin. The collagen provides the matrix for the tissue, and the smaller number of elastin fibers give elasticity and suppleness. With time, however, the amount of elastin diminishes and the collagen fibers become disorganized, cross-linking and enmeshing with each other. As a result, the tissue gradually loses elasticity. A general thinning and drying out of the skin is part of the process of aging (see Aging), and this also predisposes to wrinkling.

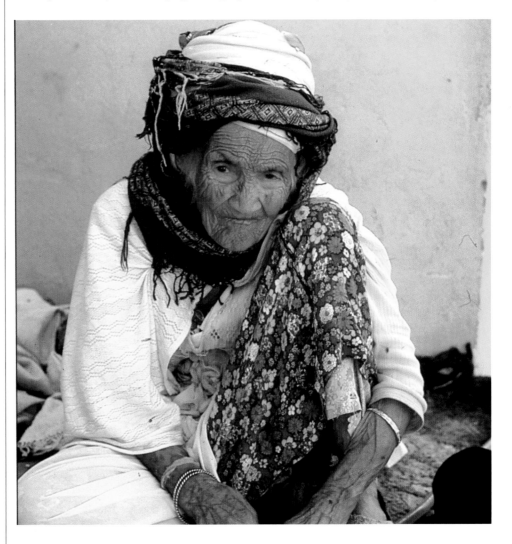

▲ *This Algerian woman is deeply wrinkled, not only from age but also because she has spent her life in a country where the sun is intensely strong for most of the year.*

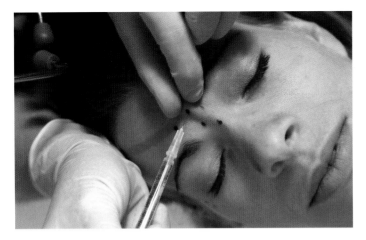

▲ *Botox injections temporarily plump out wrinkled skin for three to eight months. To achieve a smooth appearance, the injection paralyzes the muscles under the skin.*

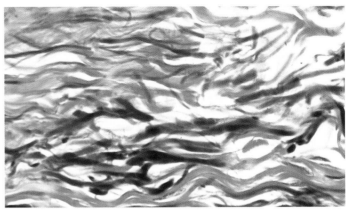

▲ *The breakdown that occurs in the skin's supportive tissue is a basic cause of wrinkling. With time, the elastin fibers (blue) diminish and the collagen fibers (pink) become loose and disorganized, resulting in loss of firmness and elasticity.*

Sunlight affects the skin (see Sunburn), and accounts for wrinkling on exposed areas of the body, particularly the face, neck, and backs of the hands. The ultraviolet component of sunlight accelerates the chemical changes in skin that cause wrinkling, and its effects are pronounced in fair-skinned people who have little natural protection against the sun's rays (see Melanin).

In the same environment, the difference between skin exposed to solar radiation and skin protected from sun is strikingly illustrated in cloistered nuns living in tropical countries. Doctors have been struck by the absence of wrinkling and other effects of sunlight on the skin of women whose dress and way of life have provided lifelong avoidance of direct sunlight.

Ultraviolet radiation has a direct effect on the DNA in the skin cells. The damage to DNA is normally repaired by natural processes of DNA repair and replication, but these are not capable of repairing all the damage, and some DNA remains abnormal. This effect is cumulative, and eventually abnormal skin is the result. This abnormality is mainly manifested in wrinkles, but it can also appear as several forms of skin cancer, including rodent ulcers (see Ulcers).

Facial expression can influence wrinkles. When someone smiles, grimaces, or frowns, furrows are formed in the skin according to which facial muscles are being contracted. Over the years these facial lines become ingrained so that they are visible all the time.

A further influence on the pattern of wrinkling is the amount and distribution of subcutaneous fat deposits in and around the face. Excess fat deposits tend to be drawn downward by gravity to form bags under the eyes, double chins, and heavy jowls. In older people, jowl creases may extend up to the cheeks, and tend to run perpendicular to the lines of facial expression, producing a crosshatch pattern of wrinkles. Finally, smoking speeds up the process of wrinkling (see Smoking), perhaps because smokers screw up their faces to prevent smoke from irritating their eyes and this grimacing accentuates the lines of expression. Also, cigarette smoke contains at least 3,000 different chemical substances, many of which are absorbed into the bloodstream and carried to every part of the body, including the skin, where they may damage the proteins of the skin .

The effects of aging cannot be put off forever, but the onset and development of wrinkles can be delayed. Perhaps the most important protective measure is to avoid prolonged exposure to hot sunshine and to use sunscreens with a high sun protection factor, which help to prevent the type of skin damage that promotes wrinkling. Dry skin has a greater tendency to wrinkle than oily skin, so using a moisturizing cream is a worthwhile preventive measure. Avoiding or cutting down on smoking may also be beneficial.

For many women, wrinkles become a particular problem around menopause, and this may be due to hormonal changes. Hormone replacement therapy may slow down wrinkling, but this is not yet proved and this therapy has other disadvantages to health (see Hormone Replacement Therapy).

There are a number of antiwrinkle creams available that vary in effectiveness. They cannot remove wrinkles but can give temporary camouflage. Some work by moisturizing and plumping up the skin; others fill in the wrinkles. The implication that collagen can be restored by skin creams should be viewed with skepticism.

Surgical treatment

Once wrinkles are established, surgical treatment is probably the only effective way of removing or reducing them, either by a face-lift or by chemical abrasion. Face-lifts (see Cosmetic Surgery) involve making incisions at the borders of the face, stretching the skin upward and outward, and restitching. The initial results are good, but wrinkling may recommence a year or two after surgery.

Cosmetic procedures to remove redundant stretched skin are not without risk. There have been cases in which too much redundant eyelid skin has been removed, with the result that the eyes have been unable to close. This quickly leads to severe exposure damage to the peripheral parts of the corneas.

In the method of chemical abrasion, a caustic gel is spread over the face and neck to break down the outer layers of skin, which are then removed with the gel. The new skin that grows in its place is usually considerably less wrinkled, but the procedure can be rather painful. Healing may take several weeks, and sometimes the skin is left looking patchily discolored.

Skin that has been treated in this way is extremely sensitive to sunlight for several weeks, and it is important to protect it and avoid ambient sunlight during this time.

See also: **Healing; Surgery**

Wrist

Questions and Answers

Doctors seem to find it difficult to find the pulse in my wrist. Why should this be?

The pulse at your wrist (the radial pulse) belongs to the radial artery. The artery may be in a slightly different position in all wrists. Your pulse may be deeper than usual or it may lie slightly to the right or left. In either case, it does not signify anything of importance, although your doctor might appreciate a warning that your pulse is difficult to find.

My wrists have always been weak. How can I strengthen them?

Why not take up a sport such as tennis or squash? Any activity in which you have to grip a racket or a club could strengthen the wrists and make them more flexible. It will have the added advantage of improving your general fitness and health at the same time.

My daughter is an avid gymnast and is always doing handstands. Could she damage her wrists?

Wrist injuries are always a risk in sports such as gymnastics, but your daughter's wrists are more likely to be strengthened than hurt. Rarely, deformities of the wrist occur as a result of exercise, but generally this happens only if the bones are already diseased or weakened.

I broke my wrist and have a cast on my arm. Can I still drive?

No. If you drive during the first few weeks you may stop the bones from mending properly. More important, you should also remember that with a cast on your arm you are a potential hazard on the road. The flexibility of your wrist will be reduced and you could be a danger both to yourself and to others.

Composed of eight bones and surrounded by tendons, the wrist is very flexible and surprisingly trouble-free. Like all bones, the wrist can break, but the most painful problems occur when the tendons become inflamed.

Each wrist is actually a complex of numerous joints between lots of little bones. This gives the joint great flexibility but makes it a potential weak spot. It is strengthened by a web of ligaments and tendons that link the bones and make lifting possible.

The structure of the wrist

The wrist is made up of eight separate bones called carpals. They are like small pebbles arranged in two rows and bound together by about twenty ligaments and tendons (see Ligaments; Tendons). The carpals sit between the metacarpals of the hand and the long bones of the arm.

The bones in the row nearest the arm, which run from the thumb to the little finger, are the scaphoid, lunate, triquetral, and pisiform. The second row consists of the trapezium, trapezoid, capitate, and hamate. The only one of these bones that is visible on the skin surface is the pisiform, which can be seen as the bumpy wrist bone.

The ligaments covering the wrist bones form a tunnel, the carpal tunnel, which prevents the long muscle tendons from springing away from the bones when the wrist is bent.

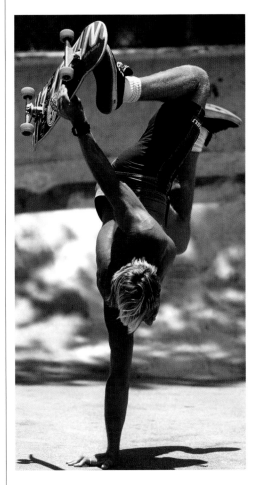

▲ *To be able to perform this action, the ligaments in the wrist must be strong enough to support the bones in the wrist.*

Movement of the wrist

The carpal joints are relatively immobile, although as a unit the wrist is very flexible indeed. The exception is the joint between the trapezium and the thumb bone. This type of joint makes it possible to grasp an object between the finger and thumb. An opposable thumb makes humans particularly adept at using tools.

Anatomically, the wrist joint is described as ellipsoid. This means that, although it enables up and down actions, side to side actions, and some circular movement, it cannot rotate like the hip and shoulder joints. This limitation helps to ensure the stability of the wrist joint. However, it is thought that the wrist joint is properly stable only when the tendons, ligaments, and muscles are acting to keep all the components of the joint in the right place. This tension is necessary, even when the body is completely at rest.

Such a fragile joint is clearly easy to damage. Lots of people will have experienced a slight sprain (see Sprains) or strain and noticed how much it affects manual manipulation—every tiny action hurts the damaged joints.

Fractures and dislocations

Of all the injuries that involve the wrist, the most common is a break at the lower end of the radius—one of the two long bones in the forearm. This is called a Colles fracture, and is

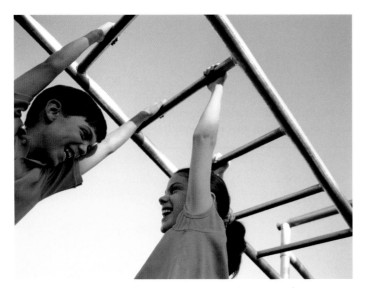

▲▼ The eight wrist bones are strengthened by ligaments and are at their most vulnerable when having to bear the brunt of the body's weight.

treated by manipulation to reset the bones and immobilization in a cast (see Fractures; Manipulation).

The small carpal bones can also suffer hairline cracks. Sometimes there is a swelling on the back of the hand, just below the thumb, but often there are no external signs, only pain and stiffness (see Stiffness) in the joint. Often even X rays do not show up these small cracks (see X Rays), but they can still be a problem. A hairline crack can separate a small portion of bone from its blood supply and this can result in bone death. If there is any suspicion that this is happening the doctor will immediately immobilize the wrist joint to prevent any more damage.

The bones of the wrist can also become dislocated if banged or moved awkwardly, especially the lunate bone in the center of the wrist and the triquetral below the little finger. The dislocation shows up as a bulge on the outside of the wrist and should be manipulated into position by a doctor as soon as possible.

Problems with the tendons

The most common problem to afflict the wrist is called carpal tunnel syndrome. The fibrous carpal tunnel encloses all the wrist bending tendons and one of the main nerves supplying the hand, the median nerve (see Nervous System). If the fibers in the tunnel become swollen or compressed they press the nerve against the wrist bones, causing pain.

The syndrome can be caused by simple overuse of the thumb and fingers. It is also common in late pregnancy when edema (swelling) can put pressure on the median nerve (see Edema; Pregnancy). It is generally more common in women than in men.

Whatever the cause, carpal tunnel syndrome begins with a sensation of pins and needles or numbness, especially in the thumb and next two fingers (see Pins and Needles). The wrist may swell up near the thumb, and the forearm and thumb are often very painful. Usually the symptoms will gradually ease as the swelling or pressure is reduced. Occasionally, however, the syndrome may be persistent or recurrent, in which case surgery may be required to effect a permanent cure.

Another problem is tenosynovitis, in which the lubricated tendon sheaths become inflamed as a result of a bacterial infection or rheumatoid arthritis. It becomes difficult and painful to uncurl the fingers, and movement may result in audible grating noises. The fingers and thumb may also feel numb as if they have permanent pins and needles. A doctor may prescribe antibiotics for bacterial infection and aspirin to relieve pain.

STRUCTURE OF THE WRIST

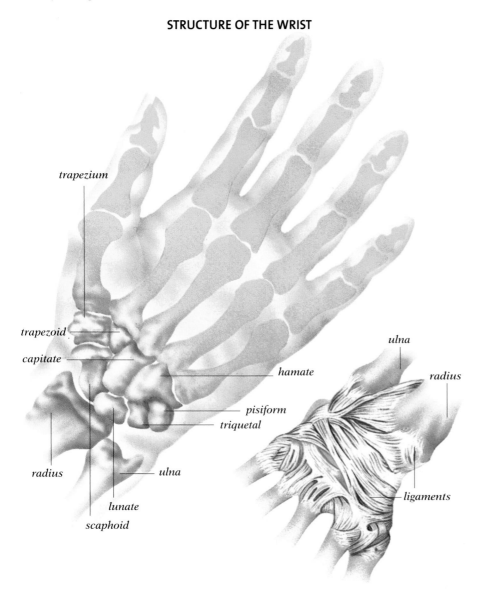

trapezium

trapezoid

capitate

hamate

pisiform

triquetal

radius

ulna

lunate

scaphoid

ulna

radius

ligaments

See also: **Carpal tunnel syndrome; Hand; Joints; Pain; Rheumatoid arthritis**

X rays

A chance discovery gave medicine one of its most valuable diagnostic tools: a window into the inside of the body known simply as X rays. Their use enables early and accurate detection of internal injury and disease.

If X rays are so dangerous, why are they still so widely used?

Modern X-ray equipment and strict safety precautions are used, and doses of X rays given in the majority of X-ray examinations are reduced to an absolute minimum. In theory, even the smallest X-ray dose carries a slight hazard, so it is a doctor's responsibility to ensure that X rays are taken only when the information obtained will be of benefit to a patient.

In the last week of pregnancy, my obstetrician said that she needed an X ray of my pelvis. Although I agreed, I worry that the X ray could have harmed my baby.

Your obstetrician was probably worried that your pelvis might have been too small for the baby to pass through safely, and was right to resolve her doubts by taking an X ray rather than risk waiting for problems to develop during labor. In this situation, an X ray was the definitive way of obtaining an answer, and worth any slight risk taken. During the first trimester the fetus is at greatest risk of damage from X rays; in late pregnancy X rays are considered relatively safe.

My brother has had many tests, and is about to have an X ray of the brain called a carotid angiogram. How is this done?

A contrast medium is injected into the carotid artery, filling the blood vessels of the brain and outlining them clearly when X rays are taken. The most comfortable and convenient way of injecting the contrast is through a long, very fine plastic catheter or tube, inserted into the femoral artery in the groin. The tube is manipulated under X-ray control until its tip lies in the artery to be studied.

On November 8, 1895, Professor Wilhelm Conrad Röntgen, while conducting an experiment at the University of Würzburg, Germany, made a chance discovery that became a legend. For the purposes of the experiment his laboratory was in total darkness, and the electrical apparatus that he was studying had been enclosed in a lightproof black cardboard cover. Yet, as he passed an electric current through his apparatus, he became aware of a faint glow coming from a piece of chemically treated paper that was lying on a nearby workbench.

Professor Röntgen had discovered how to produce invisible, mysterious rays (he named them X rays), which had not only penetrated the opaque cardboard cover but had caused the fluorescent paper to glow. Later he discovered that the rays from his apparatus could also blacken a photographic plate and produce a permanent image using the fluorescent paper. He investigated other properties of the rays and found that they could penetrate many solid objects. He placed his hand in the path of the X rays and saw for the first time an image of his own bones suddenly appear on the fluorescent paper. Today, more than 100 years later, X rays are an indispensable aid to modern diagnostic medicine (see Diagnosis), and indeed most hospitals

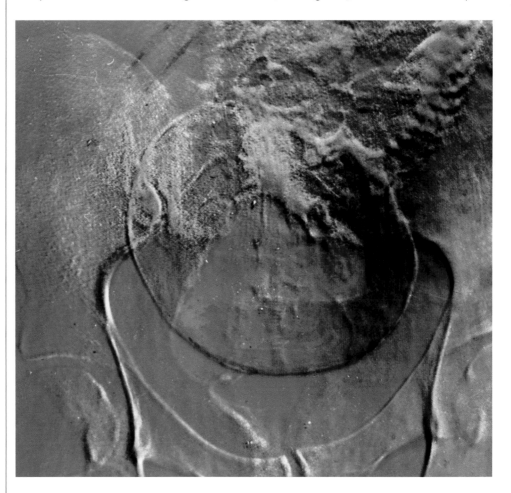

▲ *Computer color enhancement techniques add detail to X rays. Here an eight-month fetus can be seen in an ideal position, ready for birth. X rays during the last part of pregnancy are relatively safe.*

Questions and Answers

I twisted my knee months ago playing baseball. It has been troubling me ever since, and keeps locking. I'm due to have an arthrogram. What will it show?

Air and a contrast medium are injected into the knee joint under local anesthesia, giving a clear view of the joint. If you have torn a cartilage, the arthrogram will confirm this.

I hear differing opinions on the value of mammography. Is it valuable or a waste of time?

With the earlier and cruder equipment available, mammography did not much reduce the death rate from breast cancer. Now, the WHO agrees that, especially for older women, it saves many lives. With the development of high-tech full field digital mammography screening, and the use of MRI screening, we can anticipate a very high detection rate in even the earliest breast cancers.

My young daughter is to have a kidney X ray. Will it be painful, and is the dye injection risky?

In an IVU examination, an injection of a contrast medium containing iodine is given, usually into a vein in the arm. Young children understandably dislike injections, but the procedure itself will be entirely painless. Do tell the radiologist if your child has asthma, or any allergies that you know about, since an allergy to the contrast sometimes occurs.

How is it that X rays can be used to fight cancer?

X radiation can be dangerous because it damages all living cells. However, it particularly damages those cells that grow and divide profusely, as in cancer. Careful use of X rays has made it possible to destroy cancerous cells, or retard their development, while exposing healthy cells to as little radiation as possible.

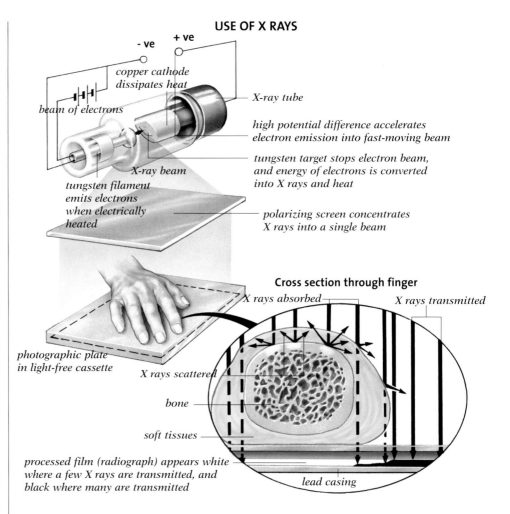

USE OF X RAYS

- ve + ve

copper cathode dissipates heat

beam of electrons

X-ray tube

high potential difference accelerates electron emission into fast-moving beam

tungsten target stops electron beam, and energy of electrons is converted into X rays and heat

X-ray beam

tungsten filament emits electrons when electrically heated

polarizing screen concentrates X rays into a single beam

Cross section through finger

X rays absorbed

X rays transmitted

photographic plate in light-free cassette

X rays scattered

bone

soft tissues

processed film (radiograph) appears white where a few X rays are transmitted, and black where many are transmitted

lead casing

▲ *X rays radiate outward from a tungsten target. They pass through the soft tissues of the body, but are absorbed by the bones. The shadow cast by the bones is caught by the photographic plate.*

spend more money on scanning departments than on any other department. The latest sophisticated technology provides a safe and reliable means of detecting disease at an early stage, and of monitoring treatment efficiently and effectively.

What are X rays?

X rays belong to the same family as light waves and radio waves, and, like radio waves, are invisible. They are produced artificially by bombarding a small tungsten target with electrons in a device called an X-ray tube. X rays travel in straight lines and radiate outward from a point on the target in all directions. In an X-ray machine, the X-ray tube is surrounded by a lead casing, except for a small aperture through which the X-ray beam emerges.

Each of the body's tissues absorbs X rays in a predictable way, and this is the property of X rays that enables them to be used in medicine to form images of the body. Bones are dense and contain calcium, which absorbs X rays well. Soft tissues, such as skin, fat, blood (see Blood), and muscle, absorb X rays much less efficiently. When, for example, an arm is placed in the path of an X-ray beam, the X rays pass readily through the soft tissues but penetrate the bones less easily; the arm casts a shadow. X rays blacken photographic film, so the shadow cast by the bones appears white, while the shadow of the soft tissues is a dark shade of gray.

The X-ray examination

An X-ray image, or radiograph, is a demonstration of the anatomy of the part of the body under examination, and it is now possible to make a detailed inspection of almost any part of the body with X rays. X rays are of greatest use in the diagnosis and follow-up of disease and disorders that alter the structure of the body. Sometimes changes in structure are so dramatic that they

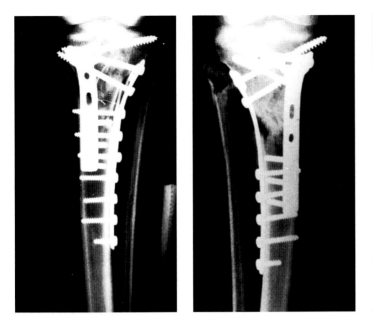

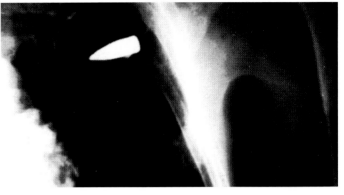

▲ *This dramatic X ray shows a bullet lodged in someone's upper chest: luckily the X ray shows no severe injury such as a punctured lung or damaged heart.*

◄ *After badly breaking both legs in a motorcycle accident, this victim had to have his bones pinned and bolted together.*

are immediately obvious even to the untrained observer, for example, in the case of broken bones (see Fractures). Frequently, however, the changes are more subtle, and may be apparent only to the trained eye of a radiologist (a doctor who specializes in the interpretation of X-ray images).

Before an X-ray examination, instructions about any special preparations that may be necessary are given to the patient when the appointment for the examination is made. In the case of examinations of the abdominal region (see Abdomen), for example, it is often preferable for the patient to take laxatives (see Laxatives) and a special diet (see Diet) for two days beforehand, since emptying the intestines results in radiographs of much improved quality.

When the patient arrives at the X-ray department, the radiographer who will be taking the X rays explains the procedure. The patient undresses to expose the area concerned, and removes any objects, such as jewelry or dentures, that might produce an image on the radiograph. The position of the patient when the X ray is taken is chosen to provide the best demonstration of the part under examination, though this position may have to be modified if the patient is sick or in severe pain. Each X-ray film is carried in a flat cassette, and the patient lies, sits, or stands so that the area of interest is in contact with the cassette. It is essential to avoid movement while an X ray is taken; movement results in a blurred image. Every effort is made, therefore, to keep the patient comfortable, to use the shortest feasible exposure time (usually a mere fraction of a second), and, if necessary, to support or immobilize the region of interest with foam pads or a cloth bandage. To take an X ray, the radiographer leaves the room and presses an exposure button on the control panel to execute the X ray. Although the control panel is situated behind a protective screen, the radiographer is still able to see and talk to the patient at all times. If it is necessary for someone to remain in the room while X rays are taken, exposure to X rays is prevented by wearing a lead apron.

Special techniques

For most purposes, a standard X-ray examination is all that is required. Special techniques are available, however, that enable areas not adequately seen on standard radiographs to be studied in greater

detail. In general, these more sophisticated techniques necessitate the use of contrast media; substances that cause the tissue concerned to become opaque. The use of contrast media (which are eliminated from the body by the kidneys) can enhance views of the gallbladder (see Gallbladder and Stones) and bile ducts, and the urinary and digestive tracts (see Digestive System). When a contrast medium is injected directly into blood vessels (a procedure known as an angiograph), the arteries (see Arteries and Artery Disease) and veins (see Veins) are clearly outlined, and any abnormalities revealed. Likewise, using a contrast medium to highlight the fluid that surrounds the spinal cord (see Spinal Cord) is useful in detecting a nerve compressed by a disk (see Slipped Disk) or by a tumor.

By using a suspension of barium sulphate (an inert, chalky mixture that is opaque to X rays), it is possible to visualize the alimentary tract throughout its length. During a barium swallow examination, the patient is given a glass of flavored barium to drink (see Barium Liquids). The patient's swallowing mechanism can be studied, abnormalities of the esophagus (see Esophagus) can be detected, and the stomach (see Stomach) is clearly outlined. During the examination, the image is viewed continuously on a monitor, and the patient lies on a tilt table so that, with careful maneuvering, each part of the stomach and duodenum can be studied in turn.

Opacification of the urinary tract is achieved by intravenous injection of a solution with iodine; this is rapidly eliminated by the kidneys. Like barium, iodine is opaque to X rays, and if X-ray films are taken at various intervals after the injection, the kidneys, ureters, and bladder are clearly shown. This technique is intravenous urography (IVU or IVP) and is of great importance in the diagnosis of many types of kidney disease (see Kidneys and Kidney Diseases).

Digital radiography

Many X-ray departments have succeeded in abandoning the use of photographic films, which caused severe storage problems and involved great expense. Digital radiography involves the use of cassettes containing, in place of film, fine-grain, reusable, scintillating screens on which images are formed by the X rays. These screens can then be scanned by a computer scanner and the images saved as digital graphics files. Or the X-ray images can be converted

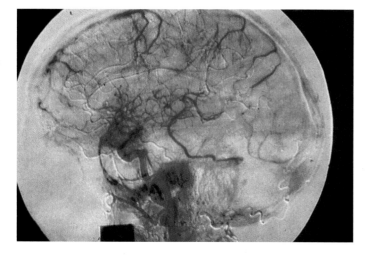

▲ *When contrast media are injected into the carotid artery, the blood vessels of the brain show up on X-ray film. The yellow band is the outline of the skull.*

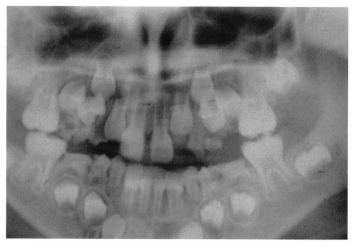

▲ *A technique called orthopantomography takes a panoramic view of the teeth: a child's second set of teeth can be seen coming through quite clearly.*

directly to graphic files. A single small hard drive can store many thousands of high-quality images that in film form would have occupied a whole room. A major additional advantage is that individual images can be called up on a computer monitor in seconds. With such systems it is also easy to make backup copies that can be stored remotely in case of loss of the originals.

Dental X rays

X-ray techniques simplify the diagnosis of a wide range of important dental problems, and are now in everyday use (see Teeth and Teething). Tooth decay can be difficult to detect, especially in the spaces between the back teeth and in other inaccessible recesses. Decay, root disease, abscesses, and infections can all be visibly demonstrated with X rays, which will confirm a diagnosis at an early stage, reveal the extent of any disease, and help determine the most suitable form of treatment. A basic X-ray examination is now a routine part of a dental checkup. The equipment used is a low-powered X-ray unit, often linked to the dentist's chair. Small films (called bitewing films) are gripped in the mouth next to the teeth to be examined. More complex conditions, such as fractures of the jaw, tumors, cysts, and problems

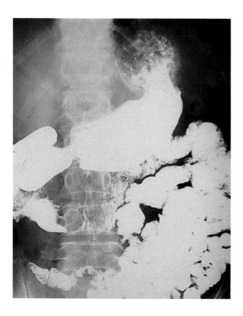

▼ *After barium liquid is swallowed, the digestive tract can be seen on an X ray. The stomach, the duodenum, and the rest of the small intestines are all shown.*

with abnormalities of growth and development of teeth, will require a much more detailed examination. A valuable technique is orthopantomography, in which an X-ray machine moves around the jaw of the patient while the X ray is taken, producing a panorama of the teeth and jaws. This technique shows both upper and lower jaws, any unerupted teeth, and the position and relationship of all the teeth on a single X-ray film.

When the two jaws do not fit together well, a side view of the face and jaws may be taken, showing the relationship of the teeth, jaws, and soft tissue. The pictures help the orthodontist to plan treatment, which may involve plates, braces, or corrective surgery (see Orthodontics).

CAT scanning

The most advanced application of X rays is computerized axial tomography, commonly known as CAT scanning or CT scanning. This is a highly sophisticated X-ray procedure developed independently by the American physicist Allan Cormack (1924–1998) and the British electrical engineer Godfrey Hounsfield (1919–); it won them jointly the 1979 Nobel Prize for physiology or medicine. The invention of the CAT scanner was one of the half-dozen most important medical advances of the 20th century.

X-ray tomography was in use long before the CAT scanner was invented. It was a method of using a swinging X-ray tube and film holder to record an image of a thin slice of the body. The results were crude, and many consecutive exposures, each involving a full dose of radiation, had to be made to provide useful information about the location and size of radiopaque objects and tissues. The major advance that made the modern CAT scanner possible was the realization that a computer could be used to store data from a large number of the separate X-ray slices and then correlate the data to synthesize a detailed image of a cross section of the inside of the body. The CAT scanner uses low-energy X-ray sources to send narrow beams of X radiation through the body to small detectors on the opposite side. These detectors are highly sensitive, and output an electrical signal that varies with the total density of the tissue through which the X rays pass. With each pulse of X rays, the resulting output from the detector is stored in a computer along

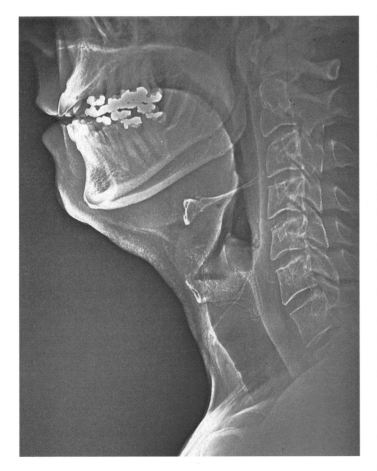

▲ *As X-ray technology advances, so the uses of X rays multiply. Special photographic techniques allow both the body outline and internal features to be captured. Here the voice box is being examined.*

with the orientation of the corresponding beam. The total radiation dose to the patient in the course of a CT scan is about the same as that of a conventional chest X ray. The computer is thus supplied with large numbers of pairs of data, the exact orientation of each of the numerous axes of X-ray projection, and, for each axis, the exact amount of attenuation caused by the bodily tissues. By solving large numbers of differential equations, the computer is able to determine the density of the tissue at every point at which the axes intersect, that is, at every point within the plane under examination.

CAT scanning provides a level of resolution and detail that was unobtainable by earlier forms of X ray, and was a major breakthrough in the noninvasive diagnosis of disease. It enables images to be made of structures, such as the brain, that are surrounded by bone. Conventional X rays are unable to show any detail in such structures. In addition, the CAT scanner has the advantage that it can show body planes in any desired orientation. The mass of data stored in the computer can be used to build up images in any required plane. Images can be viewed on a monitor screen, and records of these can be made on transparent photographic film. The basic idea behind CAT scanning has been seminal in allowing the development of a family of scanners using sources other than X rays. These include the MRI scanner (see Diagnostic Imaging), the ultrasound scanner (see Ultrasound), and the positron emission scanner (see PET Scanning).

Radiotherapy

Not only is the X-ray technique a valuable diagnostic tool; it is also an invaluable weapon against cancer. X rays can damage all living cells, but cells that are growing and dividing profusely, like cancer cells, are damaged more easily than normal cells, and are slow to recover. Radiotherapy is thus an important method of treatment in many types of cancer. Sometimes it is used on its own, as, for example, in the treatment of cervical cancer (see Cervix and Cervical Smears) or leukemia (see Leukemia), in order to destroy abnormal cells. It is also used in conjunction with other methods. For example, during the treatment of breast cancer, in which the malignant tumor is surgically removed, radiotherapy may be used to destroy any remaining tumor cells. Finally, it is used as a palliative measure (see Pain Management) to relieve symptoms of cancers too advanced to be cured. For example, in the case of cancer of the esophagus, radiotherapy may be used to facilitate swallowing, or, in the case of a brain tumor (see Brain Damage and Disease), to relieve the severity of a patient's headaches.

Both the dosage and the length of exposure take into account that radiation can also damage healthy cells. Side effects (see Side Effects) can be extremely unpleasant; they include fatigue, vomiting, and loss of hair in irradiated areas. Most side effects can be alleviated by treatment with drugs.

Some cancers are sensitive to radiotherapy, particularly tumors of the lymph glands (see Lymphatic System) and testes (see Testes), and a complete cure is often possible. The cure rate for other types of cancer is also high, depending on how early treatment is started.

Hazards of X rays

The early pioneers of radiology had no idea how dangerous excessive exposure to X rays could be, and they therefore took no precautions at all when working with X rays. They discovered to their cost that large doses of radiation cause skin burns (see Burns) and dermatitis (see Dermatitis), cataract formation in the eyes (see Cataracts), the appearance of various types of cancer, and damage to the reproductive organs resulting in genetic abnormalities in their children (see Genetics; Mutation).

Now there is a much more complete understanding of the nature of the hazards of radiotherapy, which can be reduced to a minimum. Modern X-ray film, equipment, and techniques are designed to produce high-quality images at the lowest possible radiation dose to the patient. The danger of genetic damage can be minimized by shielding the patient's reproductive organs from an X-ray beam whenever possible with a sheet of lead.

Any nonurgent X-ray examinations of women who are of childbearing age are usually carried out only during the first 10 days of the menstrual cycle (this is called the ten-day rule), during which the possibility of pregnancy is unlikely.

Outlook

With technological advances in equipment, in terms of safety and effectiveness, of both X-ray scans and radiotherapeutic equipment, most of the time benefits to patients will far outweigh any risk of serious side effects. X rays will probably continue to be an invaluable tool in modern medicine.

See also: **Bones; Muscles; Radiation sickness; Skin and skin diseases; Tumors**

Yeast infections

Many people will suffer from a yeast infection at some time in their lives. It is usually no more than a nuisance, and it presents serious problems only when associated with a severe generalized illness.

A yeast infection is caused by a fungus called candida (*Monilia*). It can affect many parts of the body, but it is particularly likely to affect the vagina. It can also occur at any time of life, from the first few weeks to old age. Normally, the infection causes little more than serious irritation, but in immune deficiency it can cause a severe general infection.

Causes

Compared with the number of bacteria that infect humans, there are very few fungi that commonly cause problems, and these fall into two groups: yeasts, the most common of which is candida; and dermatophyte fungi.

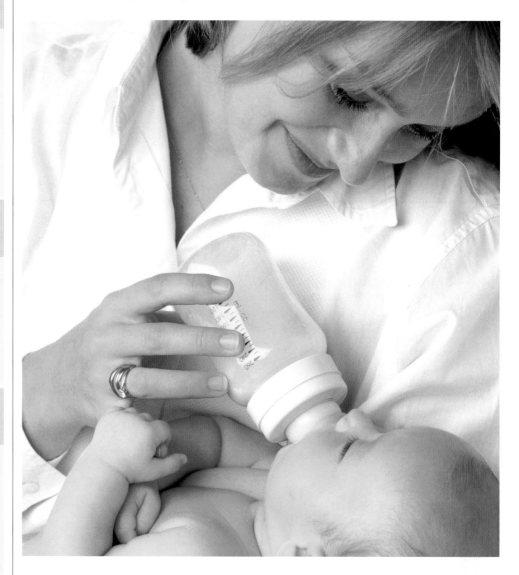

▲ *A yeast infection can occur at any time of life, even in tiny babies, although it is very unusual in breast-fed babies. Babies are most likely to get it in the mouth. An antifungal medicine will clear it up quickly.*

Questions and Answers

I am being treated for a vaginal yeast infection. Can I carry on using the pessaries when I have my period?

Yes. It is generally thought best to continue the treatment throughout the period. In fact, tampons are available that are impregnated with anti-yeast preparations.

I have athlete's foot, which I am told is caused by a fungus. How do I know it isn't thrush?

Athlete's foot is nearly always caused by one of the filamentous fungi that are best known for causing the various forms of ringworm. Thrush, however, is caused by *Candida albicans*—one of the yeast fungi. Athlete's foot can occasionally be due to candida, and this is an important factor to bear in mind if the infection is not clearing up satisfactorily.

Is it possible to prevent severe yeast infections in those very ill people who are at high risk?

There is a new practice of giving anti-candida agents by mouth to clear the gut of the infecting organisms. The gut is thought to be the source of the yeast in bloodstream infection, unless it is introduced through the skin by a medical procedure.

I have had two episodes of vaginal yeast. Does this mean that my husband keeps reinfecting me?

Candida exists everywhere that humans are, so there is no way of knowing if you are continually reinfecting yourself or getting the infection elsewhere. It may be worthwhile for your husband to be prescribed ointment to treat his penis while you treat yourself. Many doctors advise treating a woman's partner simultaneously as a matter of course.

The yeasts are very similar in form to the type of yeast that is used to make bread rise. Under the microscope they are seen as small, round organisms. It may be difficult to identify a particular candida organism. The dermatophytes are those that cause athlete's foot, ringworm, and other skin infections and feed on the flattened surface cells of the epidermis (see Ringworm; Skin and Skin Diseases).

A number of different types of candida cause disease; the most common of these is *Candida albicans* (which means white). Candida is an organism that is present on the skin or in the digestive tract of most people. If it starts to cause symptoms, this is usually because some other problem has allowed the candida organisms to multiply to a greater extent than usual.

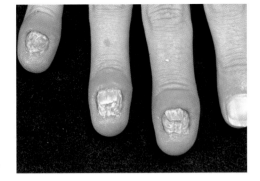

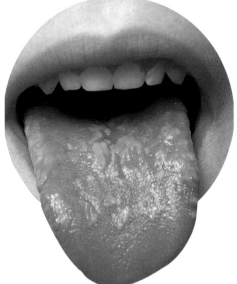

▲ ▶ *Candida fungi can cause a painful infection inside the mouth (right) and in the nail folds (above). Infection in the nail folds is most likely to happen in people who constantly immerse their hands in water, thereby weakening the protective cuticle of the nail.*

For example, elderly people often develop thrush in the mouth, and the precipitating factor is usually a cut or abrasion, perhaps where an ill-fitting denture rubs the gums or lips (see Abrasions and Cuts).

A vaginal yeast infection is the exception—it is very common for the candida organism to breed in the vagina, even if the vaginal mucosa (lining) is normal and healthy.

It is very unusual for candida to get into the body and cause systemic or deep infections (infections of the internal organs and tissues). This is most likely to happen in people who already have some illness that lowers their resistance to infection. Systemic infections may occur when patients are on drugs that suppress the immune system, or when they have a disease, such as leukemia, that has this effect (see Immune System; Immunosuppressive Drugs; Leukemia).

In rare cases, there may be a chronic infection of the mouth or vagina, or elsewhere on the surface of the body. This is called chronic mucocutaneous candidiasis. The exact cause is not certain, but it is an inherited defect in the immune system's response to disease and the problem starts in infancy or childhood.

Babies can also get thrush in the mouth any time after about the age of three weeks. This usually happens only in those babies who are bottle-fed rather than breast-fed, but it does not mean that there is anything wrong with the baby's immune system.

Symptoms

The two most common sites of candida infection are the mouth and the vulva and vagina, where infection is called vulvovaginitis. Infection in the mouth is often found in people who wear dentures, and takes the form of small white patches on the gums, on the lips, and inside the cheeks (see Dentures, Crowns, and Bridges). These may be very sore, particularly on eating, and they are usually worse in people who have a serious illness of any kind.

The yeast infection may affect large parts of the mouth and spread down into the esophagus, making eating virtually impossible (see Esophagus). This can be a definite setback for someone who is recovering from a serious operation or illness.

Vulvovaginitis as a result of yeast causes a white discharge with irritation. It can affect women of almost any age, but it seems to be most common in pregnant women and it is rare in children (see Pregnancy). Women who are diabetic are also prone to vaginal yeast infections, and it is often this symptom that initially alerts doctors to diabetes before other symptoms develop (see Diabetes).

Men can also suffer from genital candida infections. For example, inflammation of the tip of the penis (balanitis) is often caused by candida (see Inflammation; Penis and Disorders), and it is even more common for genital infection to be associated with diabetes in men than it is in women. Overall, however, candidal balanitis is less common than candidal vulvovaginitis.

Some women get vaginal yeast infections repeatedly without any predisposing condition. This problem seems to be occurring more frequently, and the conventional explanation is that these women are being repeatedly

▼ *This scanning electron micrograph (SEM) shows the* **Candida albicans** *fungus budding and forming daughter cells.*

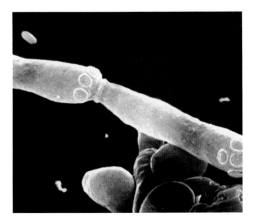

▼ *Sacs of* **Candida albicans** *fungal cells, seen in this chemical posterized image, cause yeast infections called thrush.*

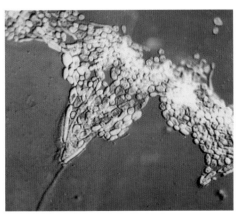

Questions and Answers

Is sex out of the question while I am being treated for a vaginal yeast infection?

Sex can be painful if you have a yeast infection, so you may prefer to abstain. However, there is no reason why you shouldn't start having sex again toward the end of a course of treatment, especially if your partner uses a condom. It is probably wise to make sure your partner is being treated too.

My two-month-old baby got a yeast infection in her mouth. I thought it was a sexually transmitted infection, but I was not having sexual relations at the time so I couldn't understand where it came from. What was the cause?

It is common for babies to get yeast infections, although they tend to occur only in those who are bottle-fed. Don't reproach yourself; it was not due to a lapse in your care. Candida fungi are so common that a baby will inevitably come into contact with one at some stage, and babies often react to their first contact by getting a mouth infection.

When my baby had a yeast infection in his mouth I found it difficult to give him the medication my doctor prescribed. Is there an easy way he could have taken it?

It can be very difficult to give medicine to small babies, especially if they lose interest in their food, as they often do with a yeast infection. Oral antifungal preparations are available for infants. Nystatin suspension, for instance, can be inserted into the fold of the cheek four to six times a day. Older children can have azole drugs such as ketoconazole or fluconazole.

Can babies get yeast infections in areas other than the mouth?

Yes, young babies can often get an infection on top of a diaper rash, since candida tends to grow in warm, moist places such as this.

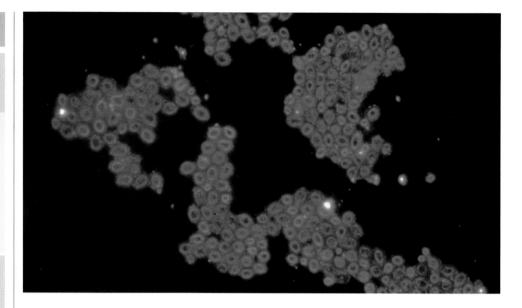

▲ *When viewed under a microscope, candida fungi appear as small, round organisms, very similar to the yeast used in making bread.*

infected, perhaps by their sexual partners. However, this is not a satisfactory theory, since candida is an organism that is present in most people most of the time, but is only occasionally the cause of symptoms. It has also been suggested that the increase in incidence of chronic vaginal yeast infections is due to the wider use of the Pill, and there is some evidence to support this view.

Other parts of the skin, including the nail folds, may also be infected. Infection of the nail folds is called paronychia or, more commonly, whitlow. *Candida paronychia* is common in people who constantly immerse their hands in water. Infection of damp sweaty skin folds also occurs.

Candida can cause infections of the internal organs in people who already have some other disease. For instance, the kidneys and urinary system may be involved in people with diabetes. Surgery can also predispose to infection, and invasive techniques, such as the use of an IV, may inadvertently introduce infection into the bloodstream (see Intravenous Infusion); the only symptom of this may be a swinging temperature. In most cases of generalized candidiasis, there is a degree of immune deficiency.

Dangers
The main danger with candida is in people who are very ill, and the more ill they are, the more likely they are to suffer from systemic infection. The most serious infections are those that affect the heart, brain, and eyes. Endocarditis (infection of the heart valves) often requires surgery to replace the affected valve, although it may also follow a valve replacement operation (see Valves), and it occurs in drug addicts.

Treatment
The treatment of simple yeast infections is effective, and differs greatly from that of systemic disease. The medications that work on surface infection—nystatin and amphotericin B—are not absorbed when taken orally. In vaginal infections, the medication is given in the form of pessaries and creams. People with recurrent mouth infections, or in whom the infection has spread into the esophagus, are given oral treatment.

Once systemic infection has been diagnosed, it is essential to use a treatment that reaches the bloodstream. The mainstay of treatment for both surface and systematic candidiasis are the azole derivative drugs, which include fluconazole, voriconazole, ketoconazole, and itraconazole.

Chronic mucocutaneous candidiasis is difficult to treat, since the defect lies with the body's ability to combat infection. The drug ketoconazole seems to be effective.

See also: Athlete's foot; Infection and infectious diseases; Mouth; Thrush; Vagina; Vaginal discharge; Vulva; Whitlow

Yellow fever

So called because it attacks the liver and causes severe jaundice, yellow fever is one of the most dangerous tropical virus diseases. It is, however, a disease that can be effectively prevented by immunization.

Yellow fever originated in West Africa but is now found in all of tropical Africa; it also occurs in Central and South America and the Caribbean. It is believed that the infection was first carried across the Atlantic during the slave trade. It does not occur in tropical parts of Asia, in North America, or in Europe, and strict controls prevent the spread of the infecting mosquito by airplane.

Causes and symptoms

Yellow fever is a disease caused by a family of viruses known as arboviruses, which are all transmitted by bloodsucking insects. Arboviruses tend either to produce symptoms of meningitis (see Meningitis), or to cause one of the hemorrhagic fevers, in which bleeding occurs into the skin and the internal organs (see Hemorrhage). Arboviruses typically infect animals as well as humans. In the case of yellow fever, monkeys and humans are the main hosts of the virus. In tropical forests, it is a major disease of monkeys, and is difficult to eliminate. Mosquitoes carry the disease from monkey to monkey, and anyone bitten by an infected mosquito can develop the disease. Apart from a cycle of infection that occurs high in the canopy of a tropical rain forest, there is also an urban cycle of infection. Thus infection may be carried directly from person to person by the infecting mosquito.

After a bite of an infecting mosquito there is an incubation period of several days while the virus multiplies in the body. Severe cases start with a sudden onset of fever (see Fevers), headache, and pain in the abdomen, back, and limbs. The patient may hemorrhage and vomit blood (see Vomiting), and because the virus injures and destroys liver cells jaundice is common (see Jaundice). The kidneys may start to transfer blood and protein into the urine. Recovery can start at any stage and if complete, confers lifelong immunity. However, in about 5 to 10 percent of cases there is a deterioration that ends in death. In some outbreaks the figure is much higher. Yellow fever can pass almost unnoticed, especially in people raised in areas where it is endemic.

Treatment

Once the disease has developed there is no curative treatment, but good nursing care helps to maintain a patient's comfort and aids eventual recovery. The outlook for patients is generally good if a fair standard of medical care is available. If the kidneys fail, for example, an intensive care unit is crucial. Relapses do not occur, and the disease confers immunity (see Immune System).

Prevention

The only preventive measure formerly available was control of the infecting mosquito. Now the major preventive measure is vaccination. An effective vaccine is available worldwide and is recommended for anyone traveling to, or through, the tropics. A certificate of vaccination is required for many countries. The vaccine provides protection from 10 days after the shot, and this lasts for about 10 years. Babies under 12 months should not be vaccinated against this disease.

▲ *Yellow fever is impossible to eradicate from the huge rain forests of the tropics, where monkeys are the hosts and mosquitoes are the carriers of the virus. Vaccination is therefore essential for anyone traveling in these regions.*

> **See also:** Bites and stings; Viruses

Questions and Answers

Is it true that you get yellow fever only from monkeys?

No. The disease has two different cycles of infection. Yellow fever is caused by an arbovirus, and it is carried from person to person by an insect. In the case of yellow fever it is the mosquito. In cities, humans are a reservoir of infection; an infected person has only to be bitten by a mosquito for the disease to be transmitted. However, in tropical forest areas, the disease primarily affects monkeys, and the cycle of infection takes place in the forest canopy where monkeys and mosquitoes live. People could catch the disease from monkeys, but only indirectly: if they were bitten by a forest mosquito.

Can you get yellow fever twice?

No. One infection provides very good immunity. People who are brought up in tropical rain forest areas do not often suffer the effects of the disease, and examination of their blood shows a high level of immunity.

Could you catch yellow fever in the United States?

Yellow fever may be brought to the United States by travelers incubating the disease, but it is unlikely to spread here. The infection has to be carried from person to person by mosquitoes, and the species of mosquito that the virus infects does not exist in the United States.

Can you be vaccinated against yellow fever?

Yes. There is an effective vaccine that is used worldwide. Vaccination is not only sometimes simply a legal requirement for anyone visiting many parts of the tropics; it is also a sensible precaution.

Yoga

I feel tense all the time. Could yoga help me relax?

Yoga could certainly help you, since it is aimed at relaxing both body and mind. The asanas, or postures, are performed slowly and gracefully, so the mind is soothed while the body is exercised. Breathing exercises and relaxation and corpse postures are good for relieving tension. You may benefit after only a few sessions.

Yoga postures in books look so difficult I'm sure I couldn't do them. Is this what yoga is about?

No. What you have seen are postures for advanced students. There is a wide range of simple and graceful exercises for beginners. With practice you will find your body becoming more supple and you will be able to get into postures you would once have thought impossible.

My husband says I am too old at 61 to take up yoga. Is he correct?

No. Many people in their sixties practice yoga; but check with your doctor beforehand, then join a class and practice daily. Yoga exercises are ideal for older people because they are carried out slowly: you ease your body into a position rather than forcing it. Yoga will help you feel lighter on your feet, more alert, and more relaxed.

Can I lose weight by taking up yoga exercise?

Yoga alone may not cause you to shed many pounds, but you should look and feel more trim because yoga exercises firm and tone the muscles. Go on a diet when you take up yoga. Yoga postures firm up the abdomen, upper arms, and thighs, which are prone to flabbiness if you are dieting.

To someone who has never tried yoga, it may appear to be exercise that is difficult to perform. In fact, yoga is exercise that gradually progresses; and it has been proved to be both physically and mentally beneficial.

The word "yoga" means union or fusion. Yoga is a system of physical and mental control based on a philosophy that originated in India. It grew out of the belief that a human being should strive to merge his or her spirit with the universal spirit, or a transcendental consciousness.

The philosophers believed that this union could be achieved through physical and mental discipline and that this discipline would eventually lead the individual toward total identification with this higher consciousness.

In the form most often practiced in the West, however, yoga is basically a series of exercises or postures that relax the mind and body, and emphasize harmonious coordination of movement, stretching, and breathing. While achieving these aims, yoga exercises also help to tone up muscles, stimulate blood circulation, regulate digestive processes, and improve mental equilibrium. Equally important, yoga can be mastered by anyone with the right motivation.

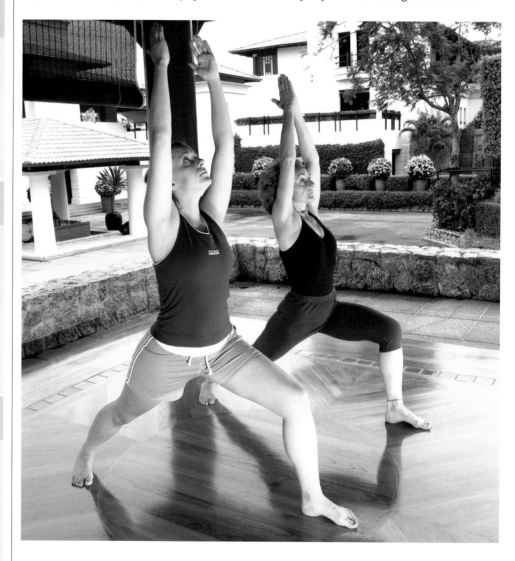

▲ *Practicing yoga exercises by the sea or in the open air can induce a healthy feeling of well-being and relaxation.*

Yoga and health

Yoga exercises comprise a series of body-stretching postures that are intended to work on the whole body. The postures are performed slowly, gracefully, and thoughtfully to achieve serenity of mind as well as physical health and flexibility. Regulated breathing exercises are usually part of the program.

The discipline of yoga requires practice, but the rewards are quickly apparent. Even a beginner will get a feeling of well-being from postures intended to exercise every tendon, muscle, and ligament. Because there are no quick or jerky movements, yoga is ideal for students from age seven to 70. However, anyone suffering from a medical condition should consult his or her doctor before taking up the discipline.

Each exercise, whether simple or complicated, is designed to benefit a different area of the body. The postures are executed slowly and then held for a period of time to allow the muscles a chance to derive the maximum benefit from the position. The contortions that many people associate with yoga are for advanced students only.

Not only are the muscles toned and firmed by yoga, but the internal organs also benefit. For example, abdominal exercises produce taut muscles and stimulate and relax the abdominal organs. Similarly, inverted positions benefit the heart and the lungs while increasing the supply of blood to the brain. The result is that many people find that they are less fatigued and more alert after a session of yoga than they were before.

Special breathing techniques are often used in conjunction with the physical yoga exercises. The basis of yoga breathing is a deeply drawn-in breath, filling the lungs and pushing the stomach out like a balloon. This is held for a few seconds and then released slowly, while the person is contracting the stomach. Breathing is done through the nose, and slow, deep breaths of this kind also help to release stress and tension (see Tension).

Yoga and dieting

Many people associate yoga with particular types of diet, such as vegetarianism. It is not necessary for people to change their diet to perform yoga, although serious students do not usually eat much heavy, rich food because it can interfere with performing the more complicated exercises.

Yoga alone will probably not induce any great weight loss, but there may be a dramatic improvement in appearance, since the exercises firm up the muscles and improve posture. For overweight people yoga should, ideally, be combined with a diet, since it will keep the body firm even as the individual loses weight. Diet without exercise can result in folds of flabby skin. Yoga exercises are particularly useful in that they work on every part of the body, including the abdominal area, the upper arms, and the thighs—areas that are prone to flabbiness.

While it is true that an Indian yogi would be a vegetarian, yoga as a philosophy stresses moderation. The Indian yogi abstains from meat because it is hard to digest, but this is not necessary for everyone. For good health, a diet low in refined sugars and starch, a minimum of canned or frozen foods, and an emphasis on whole wheat bread, milk, dairy products, fresh vegetables, and fresh fruit will combine well with yoga exercises (see Diet).

Yoga practice demands that food should be well-chewed as an aid to digestion and that, ideally, the stomach should be only half full at the end of each meal; this allows the digestive juices to

---

Yoga breathing exercises

Ideally, yoga breathing exercises should be performed before starting the postures. They are not hard to master and are of great value in calming the mind, relaxing the system, and combating fatigue. The complete breath can be practiced in any spare moments. All the exercises can be performed either sitting or standing.

Abdominal breath: 1. Place your hands lightly on your abdomen. 2. Inhale slowly and deeply through the nostrils, pushing your stomach out like a balloon. 3. Exhale slowly through the nose, contracting the abdomen. 4. Repeat three times.

Bellows breath: 1. Place your hands on your rib cage. 2. Inhale slowly and deeply, expanding the ribs sideways. 3. Exhale slowly, contracting the rib cage. 4. Repeat three times.

Clavicular breath: 1. Place your fingers on the clavicular area above the chest. 2. Inhale slowly and deeply, and feel the back of your throat fill with air. 3. Exhale slowly. 4. Repeat three times.

Complete breath: This combines the three previous exercises. 1. Exhale; then, while counting up to eight, inhale deeply, raising your shoulders, pushing out your abdomen and expanding your rib cage. 2. Hold your breath while counting up to eight. 3. Exhale slowly counting up to eight. 4. Pause for 10 seconds, then repeat.

Alternate nostril breathing: 1. Close your right nostril with your right thumb. 2. Inhale slowly and deeply through your left nostril. 3. Now close your left nostril with two fingers. 4. Hold your breath for two seconds. 5. Take away your right thumb, opening your right nostril and exhaling through it. 6. Repeat by inhaling through the left nostril and exhaling through the right. 7. Repeat the whole exercise three times.

To perform these exercises correctly, there are a few points you should remember. Always exhale as slowly as you inhale—don't let your breath out in a rush. Always take as deep a breath as you can, and always empty the lungs fully. This is designed to bring as much oxygen as possible into the system.

---

function efficiently. This is good practice for everyone, particularly anyone who suffers from digestive disorders.

Medical conditions

Many people have reported gaining relief from a wide range of medical conditions by practicing yoga and, while it is difficult to verify these claims with any accuracy, there are certain exercises that do seem to benefit people suffering from specific complaints.

The abdominal exercises, like the Cobra and the Bow, help all the organs of the digestive system to function without the aid of laxatives. These exercises are claimed to alleviate conditions such as indigestion, constipation, heartburn, and even colitis. The positions

Questions and Answers

I've had a baby and feel flabby. Could yoga help me firm up?

Yes. Yoga exercises are excellent because they tone all the muscles of the body. Check with your doctor first and, as long as he or she has no objection, join a yoga class and practice daily. If you feel particularly flabby around the abdominal region, ask your yoga teacher to show you the specific exercises for this area. You can then practice them as often as you like. Don't overstrain your body in your eagerness to get your figure back; yoga is a gentle art, and you will soon see results.

My eight-year-old daughter wants to take up yoga. Is she too young?

No. Her youthful flexibility will give her a great advantage. The exercises will teach her body control, concentration, gracefulness, and the ability to relax. She will probably progress fast and soon be able to master complicated postures.

I suffer from backaches. Could yoga help?

Possibly, but check with your doctor before joining a class. Some yoga postures are particularly helpful to sufferers from backache, lower-back pain, and rheumatism. Explain the problem to your teacher and ask him or her to teach you postures that might help you most.

My friend claims that since taking up yoga she feels better, eats less, and sleeps more soundly. Are her claims correct?

Almost everybody who takes up yoga exercises and practices them regularly reports an improvement in physical and mental well-being, so your friend could be correct in attributing her good health to yoga. Why not put it to the test? Ask your friend if you can accompany her to the classes and find out for yourself what the benefits are.

The Soorya Namaskar or sun salutation is performed at the start of each session of yoga. It consists of a cycle of gentle, almost langorous, postures, which loosen up all the muscles that will come into use, and promote a serene state of mind.

G

A

B

C

F

D

A selection of yoga exercises, each of which has a specific aim or benefit. Some are easy; others are more difficult, and should be attempted only when a yoga teacher feels that his or her pupil is ready. Clockwise, from top to bottom: the Cobra (A) is an effective abdominal exercise; the Locust (B) works on the spine; the Bridge (C) benefits the back; the Wheel (D) is a spectacular posture that attacks the areas where fat tends to accumulate; the Plow (E) is a fine exercise for relieving backache; the Bow (F) is a posture especially suited to the dieter's needs; and, finally, the headstand with legs extended (G; opposite page) strengthens the heart and improves blood circulation.

E

Yoga relaxation

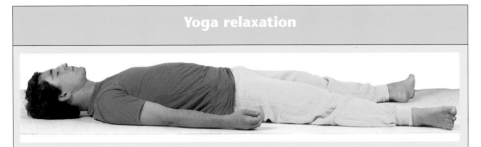

Always end a session of exercises with the relaxation or corpse posture. It can also be performed on its own whenever you have the free time or opportunity. Carried out correctly—and it does take practice—it relaxes mind and body, easing tension, reducing fatigue, and producing a feeling of revitalization.

Lie on your back on the floor, arms by your side, legs straight out and together. Try to let go completely, imagining that your body has great weight and is sinking through the floor. Try to empty your mind of all thoughts except the weight of your body. Now tense, then relax every part of your body in turn in this order:

1. The scalp and the forehead. 2. Eyes and eyeballs. 3. Mouth and jaw. 4. Throat. 5. Neck. 6. Shoulders. 7. Thorax. 8. Upper arms. 9. Forearms. 10. Hands and fingers. 11. Abdomen. 12. Buttocks. 13. Thighs. 14. Calves. 15. Feet and toes.

Lie for one minute, then repeat, starting with feet and toes. Lie flat again for one minute. Sit up slowly. Rise slowly.

that exercise the spine, such as the Locust, Plow, Tree, or Bow, or back stretching, help to relieve backache, menstrual cramps or other cramps, lower-back pain, and rheumatism. Inverted positions, such as the headstand and shoulder stand, strengthen the heart and allow blood to flow freely to the organs in the upper parts of the body; they can also help sufferers from ailments such as asthma or bronchitis. In addition, these inverted positions also result in increased circulation to the thyroid gland, and stimulate its function in regulating the body's metabolism and increasing an overall feeling of vitality (see Thyroid).

For people who are obese, exercises that may be helpful include the Bow, knee and head, back stretching, Twist, and Triangle. These exercises attack areas where fat tends to accumulate and, when combined with a sensible diet, can bring about a marked improvement (see Obesity).

Some yoga exercises can be continued through the first months of pregnancy, although a doctor's opinion should be sought. Some postures—the headstand, for example—are not recommended, but some of the simpler exercises can be very beneficial. After pregnancy, after consultation with a doctor, yoga can be resumed and can be

effective in firming up abdominal muscles and toning up the body. Many breathing exercises used in natural childbirth are derived from yoga breathing techniques.

The mental tranquillity that ensues is another benefit of yoga, and helps to ensure sound sleep. Many people report that yoga cures their insomnia (see Insomnia). Increased mental alertness and clarity of mind are also noticed. Converts to yoga say they can carry out daily tasks with less fatigue than before.

Rejuvenation

In India many yogis live to an advanced age, and while this may be due in part to their diet, yoga exercises are probably also influential. Yoga cannot arrest the process of aging, but it can keep a person looking younger for longer.

Yoga can be taken up by people in their sixties and seventies—though they should discuss their intention with a doctor before doing so—since the exercises do not force the body in any way.

With practice, the stiffness that is common in later life can be replaced by a degree of suppleness. It has also been claimed that yoga helps to relieve arthritis, which for many people is the bane of old age (see Arthritis). Certainly more elderly people should feel the benefits of increased flexibility of muscles, better posture, increased vigor, and alertness.

Many older people suffer from insomnia, and this can be alleviated by yoga. Many will also benefit from postures that ease backache and rheumatism.

Yoga classes are held all over the United States, so it should not be difficult to locate a class in a certain area. Many cities offer yoga holidays of weekends or longer.

▶ *Yoga is ideal exercise in middle and old age, since the postures are effected smoothly and do not force the body at all.*

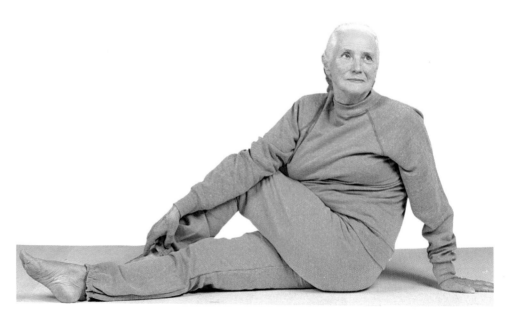

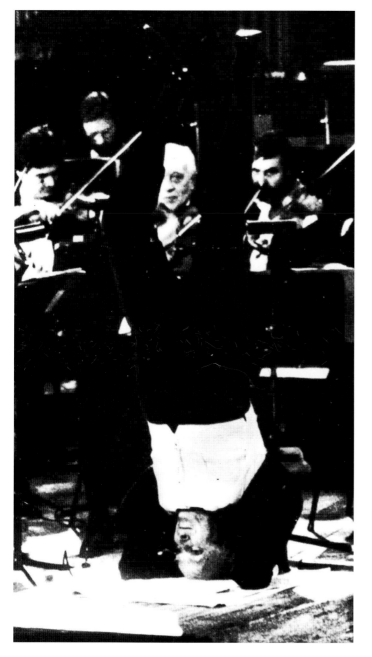

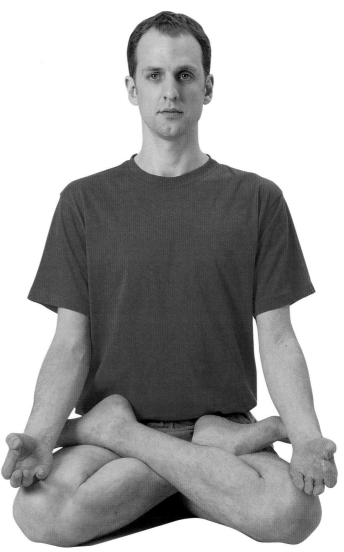

▲ *Yehudi Menuhin, violinist and conductor, was a fervent disciple of yoga. Here he conducted the centenary concert of the Berlin Philharmonic standing on his head.*

▲ *The lotus position is probably one of the best-known yoga poses. It is a meditation posture that helps to create serenity of mind and a feeling of well-being.*

A local library or community center can usually provide details about yoga classes. It is better to learn in a class, since a teacher will be able to monitor progress better than people can themselves, and he or she will be able to introduce students to new exercises as they become ready.

Once people have started their classes, however, they need to practice daily for best results. Yoga exercise should not be carried out within two hours of eating a meal, and constricting clothing should not be worn while a person is doing the exercises. A large space is not necessary, but it helps to practice in front of a mirror.

A daily routine could be the exercises that have been learned in class. Remember that each pose should be started and finished slowly. For best results yoga students should try to exercise for at least 15 minutes daily; the time of day is unimportant. When someone first starts yoga exercises he or she will probably find that the body is very stiff and does not respond well to commands. The stiffness will disappear with practice and he or she will soon find it possible to take up postures that once looked impossible. One of the benefits of yoga is that just attempting an exercise, even if it cannot be completed, can benefit the body. The key to success is not to feel discouraged after one or two failures; if someone is willing to persevere, he or she will soon feel the benefits.

See also: **Alternative medicine; Anxiety; Breathing; Exercise; Relaxation; Stress; Stress management; Wellness; Zest**

Zest

Questions and Answers

An eager relish to get the most from life, a lively will to tackle its problems— zest is an aspect of people's well-being, largely determined by personality type and genetic inheritance, that fluctuates with their health and state of mind.

I don't sleep as well as I used to. This situation leaves me tired and irritable during the day, and I don't have the zest for life that I once had. What can I do?

Try to find out what is interfering with your sleep. Perhaps you are subconsciously depressed or anxious about something. Perhaps you are not getting enough leisure time, so that you take work worries to bed with you. If you can't resolve the problem yourself within two weeks, ask your doctor for help. However, don't start taking sleeping drugs, which may end up by making the situation worse.

I feel very sluggish these days. Would vitamin pills help?

No, probably not. You must first find out why you are less full of life than you used to be. It could be something physical, such as anemia. However, it might equally be something mental, like a nagging worry or unresolved problem. If necessary, get your doctor to help sort it out with you.

Since my husband died I have become miserable. I used to be such a lively person. Will I ever get back my zest for living?

Yes, you will eventually. Grief and bereavement are very draining, and you are unlikely to feel much zest for anything while grief remains with you. Although grief is a very natural thing, it can sometimes go on longer than is really necessary—it becomes a kind of habit. Perhaps you need to give yourself a better chance to get out of it by mixing more with other people, going to parties, and so on, even if you don't feel much like doing so at first. Buy yourself some new clothes; try doing something different or going somewhere completely new. It's surprising how quickly things can change once you make the first all-important move.

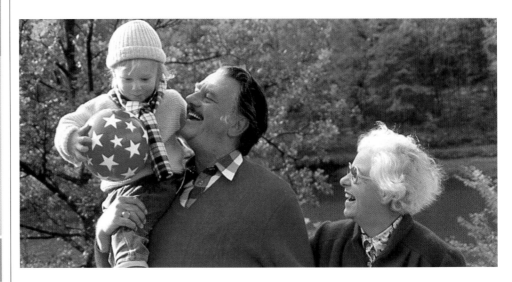

▲ *Zest for living, which allows people to draw vitality from nature and those around them, need never desert them. Grandchildren can be a source of inspiration for the elderly.*

Strictly speaking, "zest" is not a medical term, but it is a word used by both doctor and patient when discussing lethargy, depression, illness, or even behavior or attitude. The term "zest" means great interest, keen enjoyment, and an enthusiastic relish for life. Zest is not something all people have or even should have, but when it is missing from a normally lively person it may be cause for concern.

Physical well-being

A loss of zest may be symptomatic of impending sickness, anxiety, depression, or even poor eating habits or excessive living (see Anxiety). If a person feels that his or her zest for life has disappeared, then it is time to sit back and take stock. Is a balanced diet being enjoyed, or has sluggishness come about through overindulgence and lack of exercise? What about alcohol? It is easy to get into a state of subintoxication in which the brain is seldom free from the numbing effects of alcohol (see Alcoholism). Even sleeping pills and tranquilizers can dampen a person's energy if taken on a regular basis, and the most lively of people may find their joie de vivre waning (see Tranquilizers). A temporary course of drugs such as antibiotics may have a similar effect (see Antibiotics).

Regular sleep and exercise, plenty of play, and a vacation (at least once a year) involving a complete change of scene are important if a person is going to keep his or her energy levels high.

All in the mind

Of course, sickness and bereavement do drain a person's resources, and it often takes much time and adjustment before zest for life returns (see Grief). However, zest is not just a matter of physical condition and enthusiasm; it is very much a state of mind. If a person's lifestyle is flat, excitement is missing, or work is boring and undemanding, then this may affect the mental and emotional state, producing an attitude of bored indifference. Only by objectively assessing all aspects of the life can one determine those aspects of it that need changing. Once the first steps have been made, zest may return fairly quickly. However, there may be a medical cause behind the loss of zest, so this should be discussed with a doctor. Simply talking it through may be all that is needed.

See also: **Depression; Exercise; Lethargy**

INDEX

Headings and page numbers in **bold** refer to complete articles. Page numbers in *italics* refer to illustrations or their captions.

Index